DEAR READER,

THIS BOOK IS A PRODUCT OF MY DECADES-LONG PASSION FOR EXPERIMENTAL DIGITAL ART.

I USED A COMBINATION OF HAND-DRAWN DESIGNS, DALLE-3 GENERATIVE AI, AND POST PRODUCTION IN PHOTOSHOP AND ADOBE ILLUSTRATOR TO ACHIEVE THE IMAGES IN THIS BOOK.

THE ADVENT OF VISUAL GENERATIVE AI IS A MAGNIFICENT WORLD OF CREATIVITY, EXPLORATION AND OPPORTUNITY FOR ARTISTS. I HOPE THIS BOOK INSPIRES YOUR OWN USE OF AI TO UNLEASH YOUR CREATIVITY!

AS A DIGITAL ARTIST FOR OVER 25 YEARS, I REALIZED THAT GENERATIVE AI OPENS A NEW WORLD OF CREATIVE POSSIBILITIES.

I WANTED TO CREATE A BOOK WITH ART THAT VISUALLY STIMULATE THE MIND, ENTERTAINS AND BRINGS SMILES TO FACES.

BY COLLABORATING WITH AI, I WAS ABLE TO MAKE MY VISION COME TO LIFE. I TOOK GREAT DELIGHT IN CREATING THIS BOOK, AND I HOPE YOU WILL BE DELIGHTED BY READING IT.

SINCERELY, 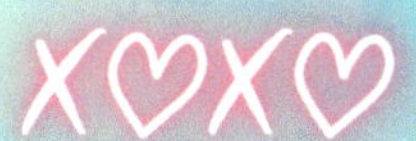

Carlie Partridge

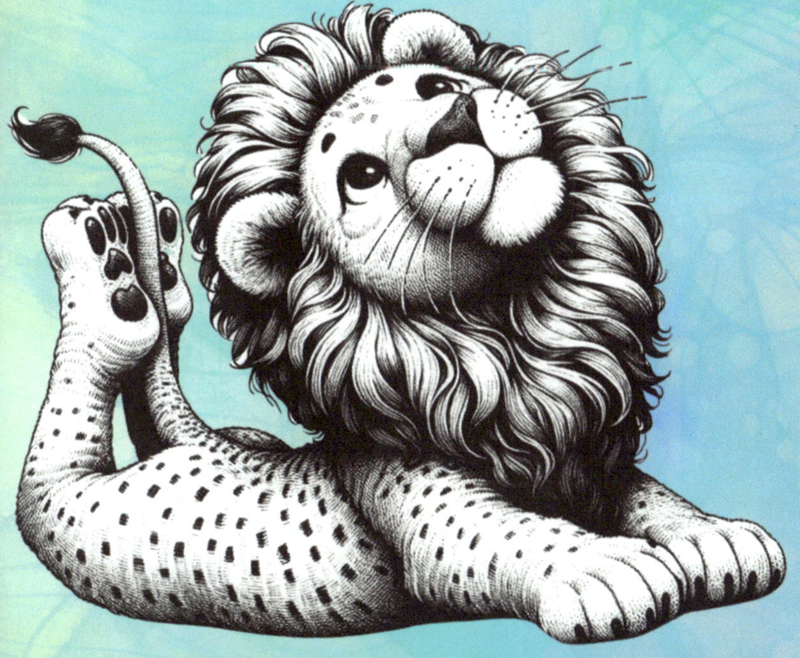

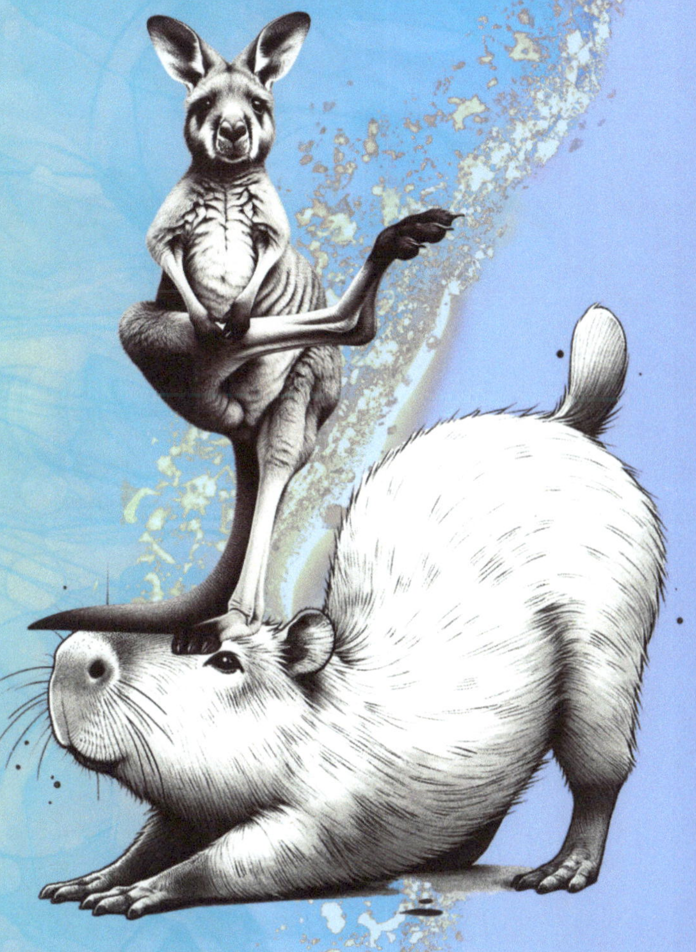

DEDICATION

This book is dedicated to the most kind and creative children in my life:

SCARLETT

HAZEL

ABRAHAM

&

WESLEY

XOXO

Carlie Partridge

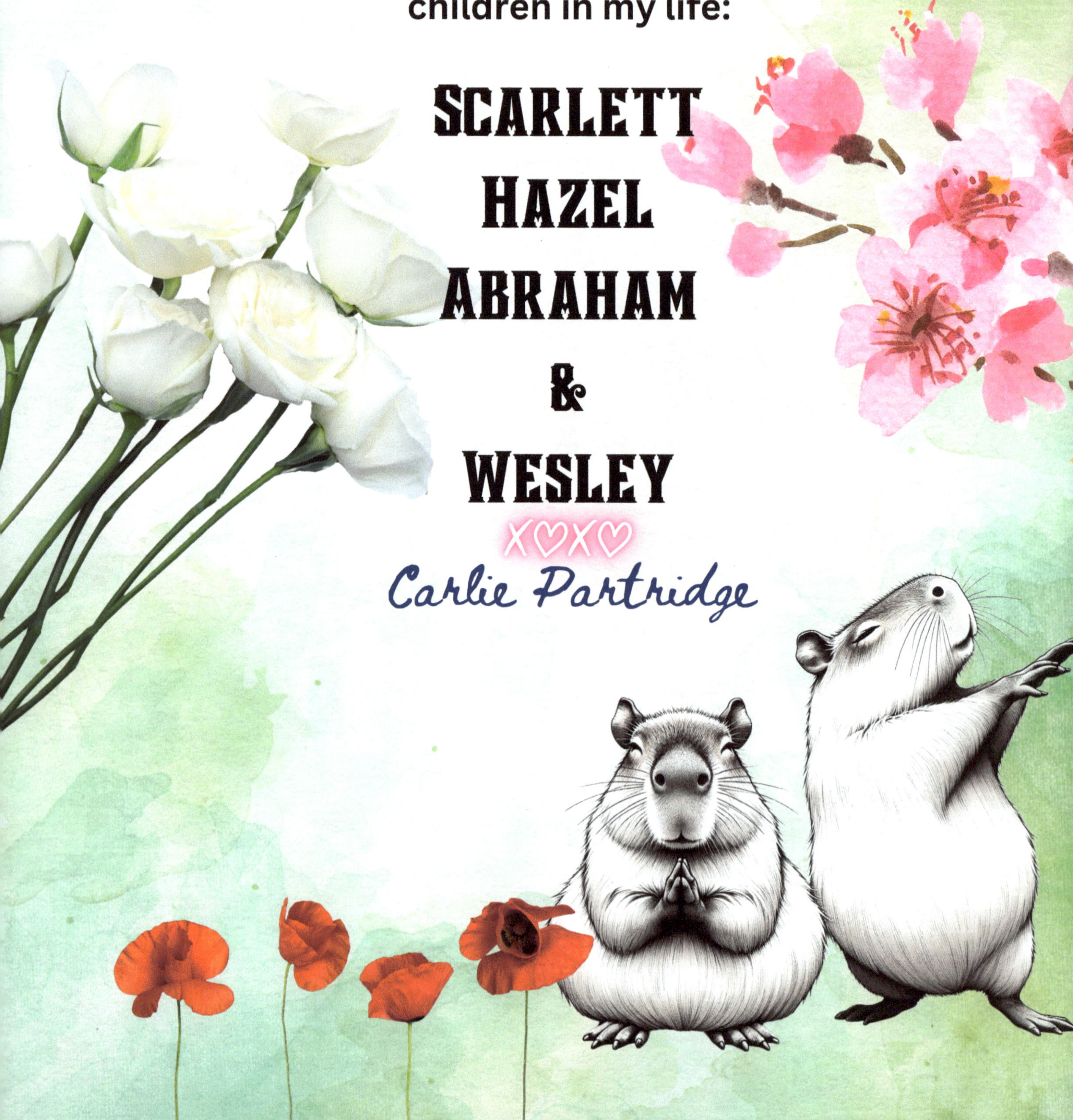

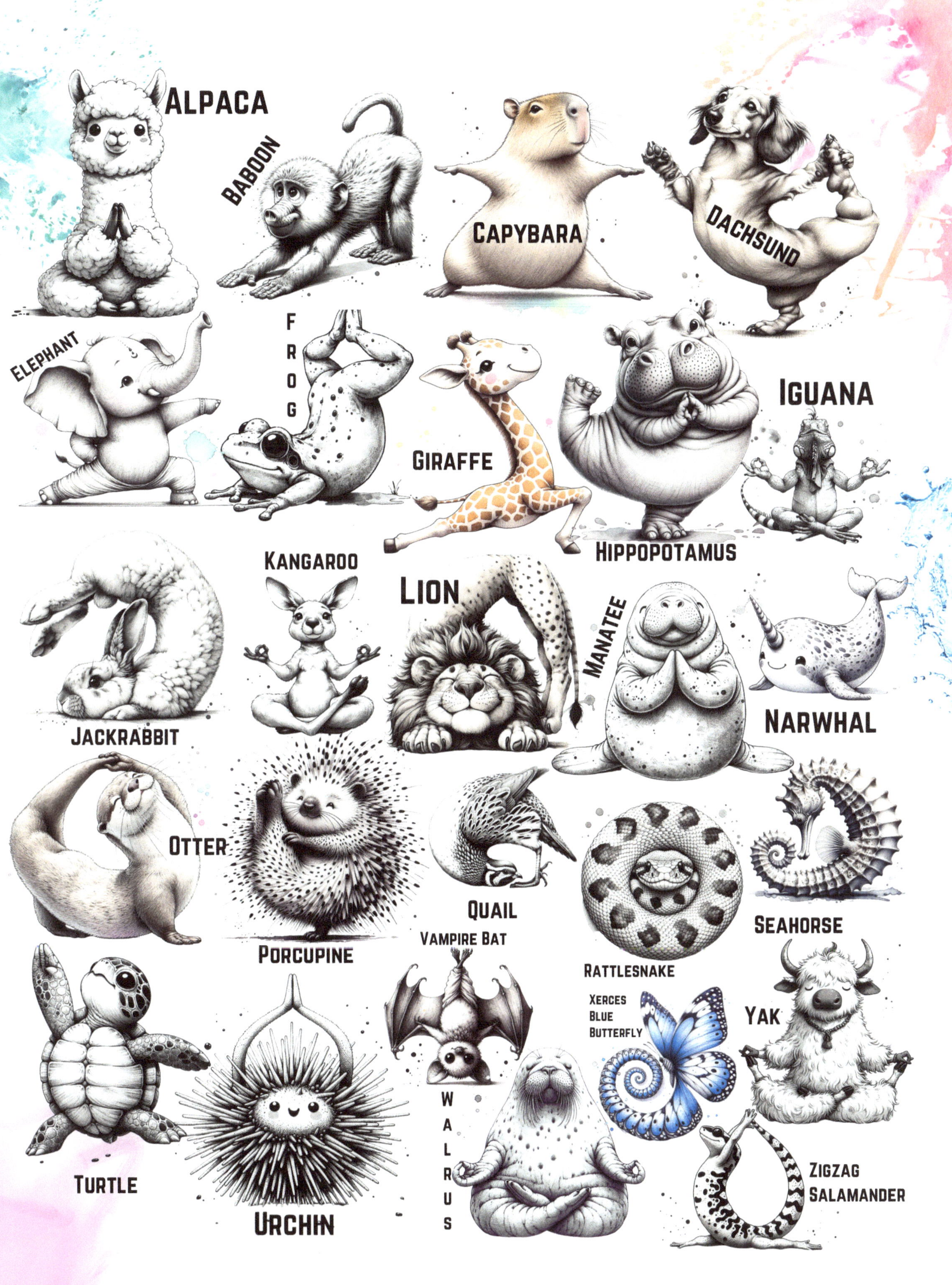
Alpaca
Baboon
Capybara
Dachsund
Elephant
Frog
Giraffe
Hippopotamus
Iguana
Jackrabbit
Kangaroo
Lion
Manatee
Narwhal
Otter
Porcupine
Quail
Rattlesnake
Seahorse
Turtle
Urchin
Vampire Bat
Walrus
Xerces Blue Butterfly
Yak
Zigzag Salamander

ALPACAS ARE RELATED TO CAMELS, BUT THEY ARE SMALLER AND FLUFFIER.

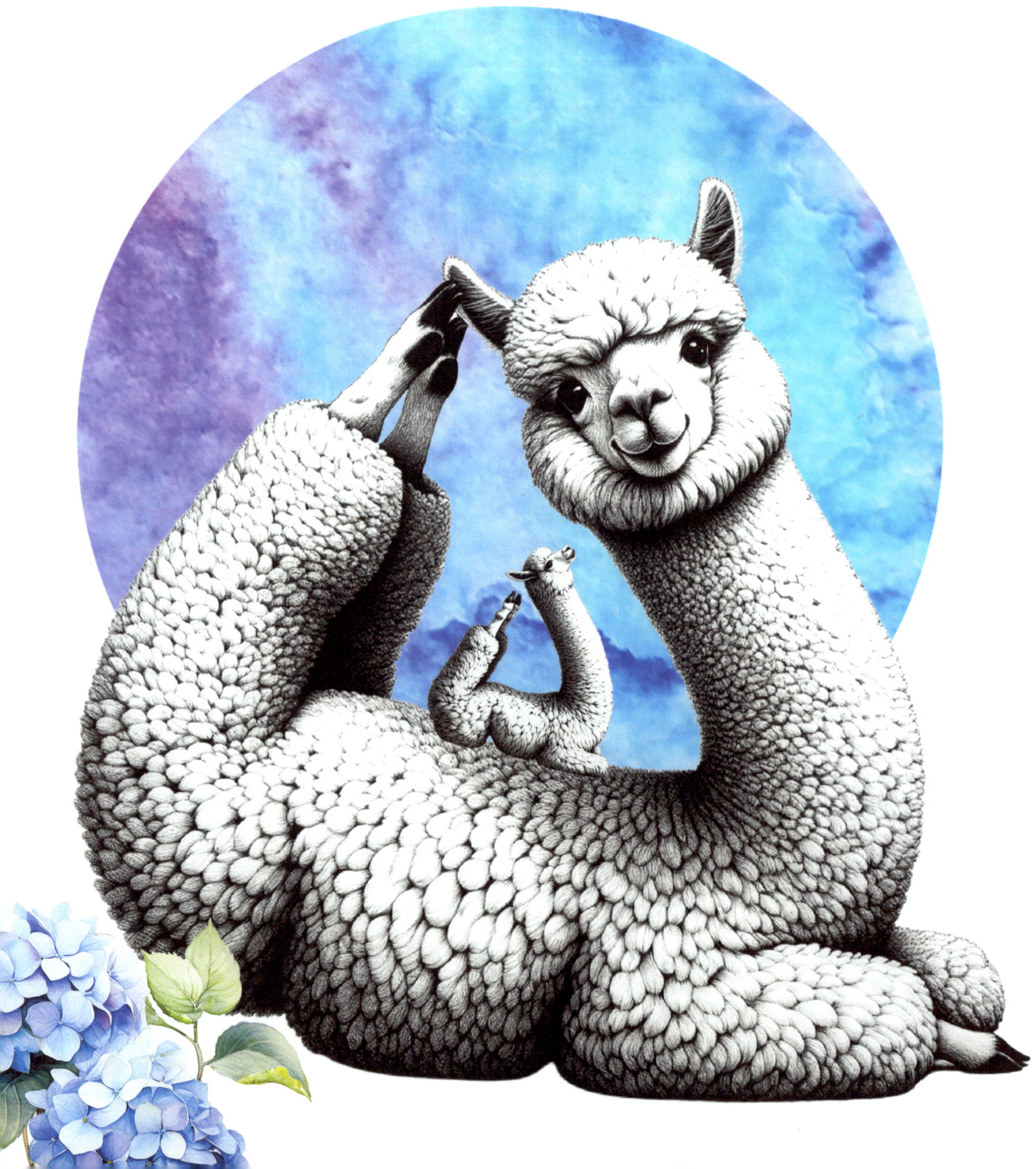

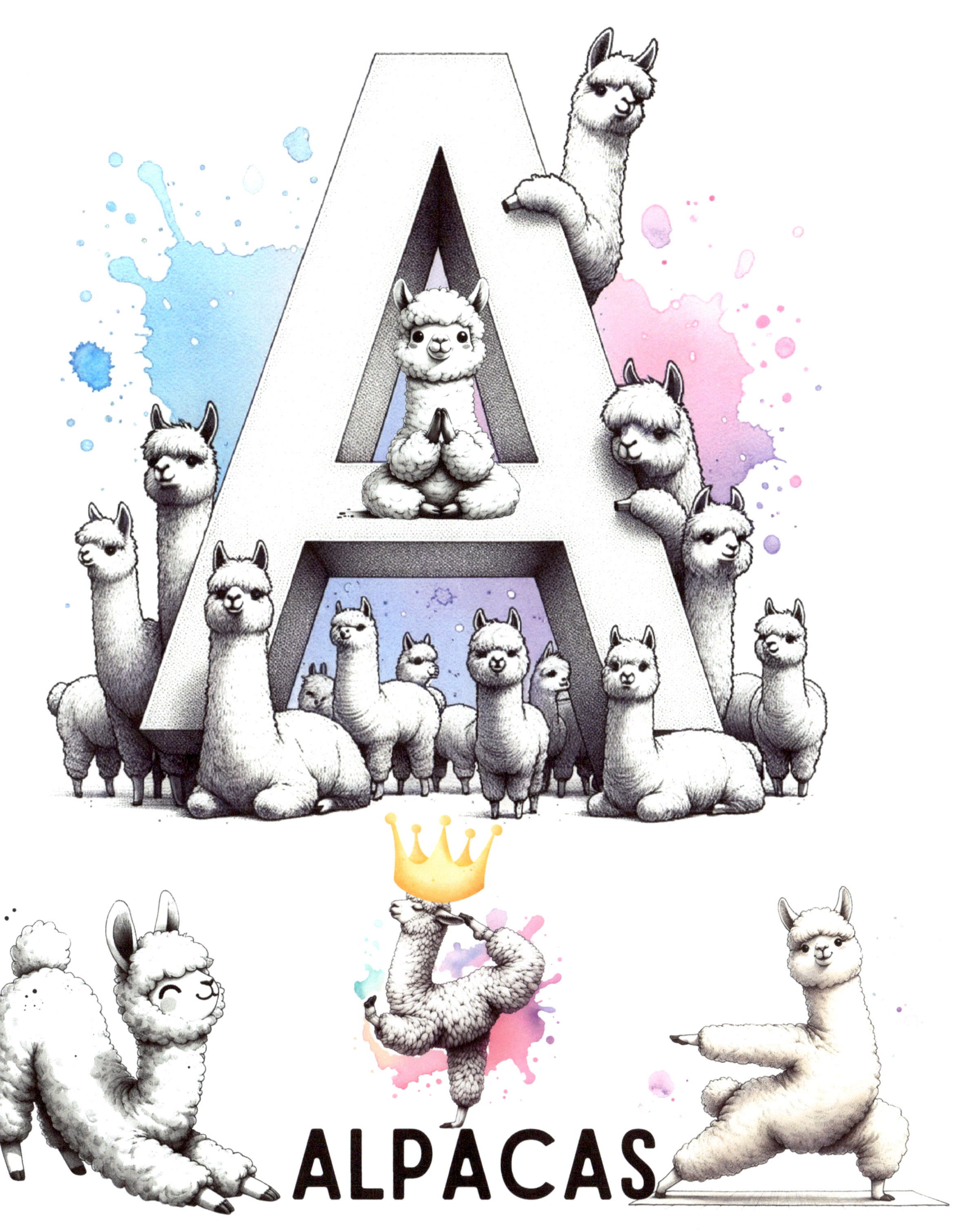

ALPACAS

BABOONS ARE THE WORLD'S LARGEST MONKEYS. AND THE OLDEST. THEY HAVE EXISTED FOR OVER TWO MILLION YEARS.

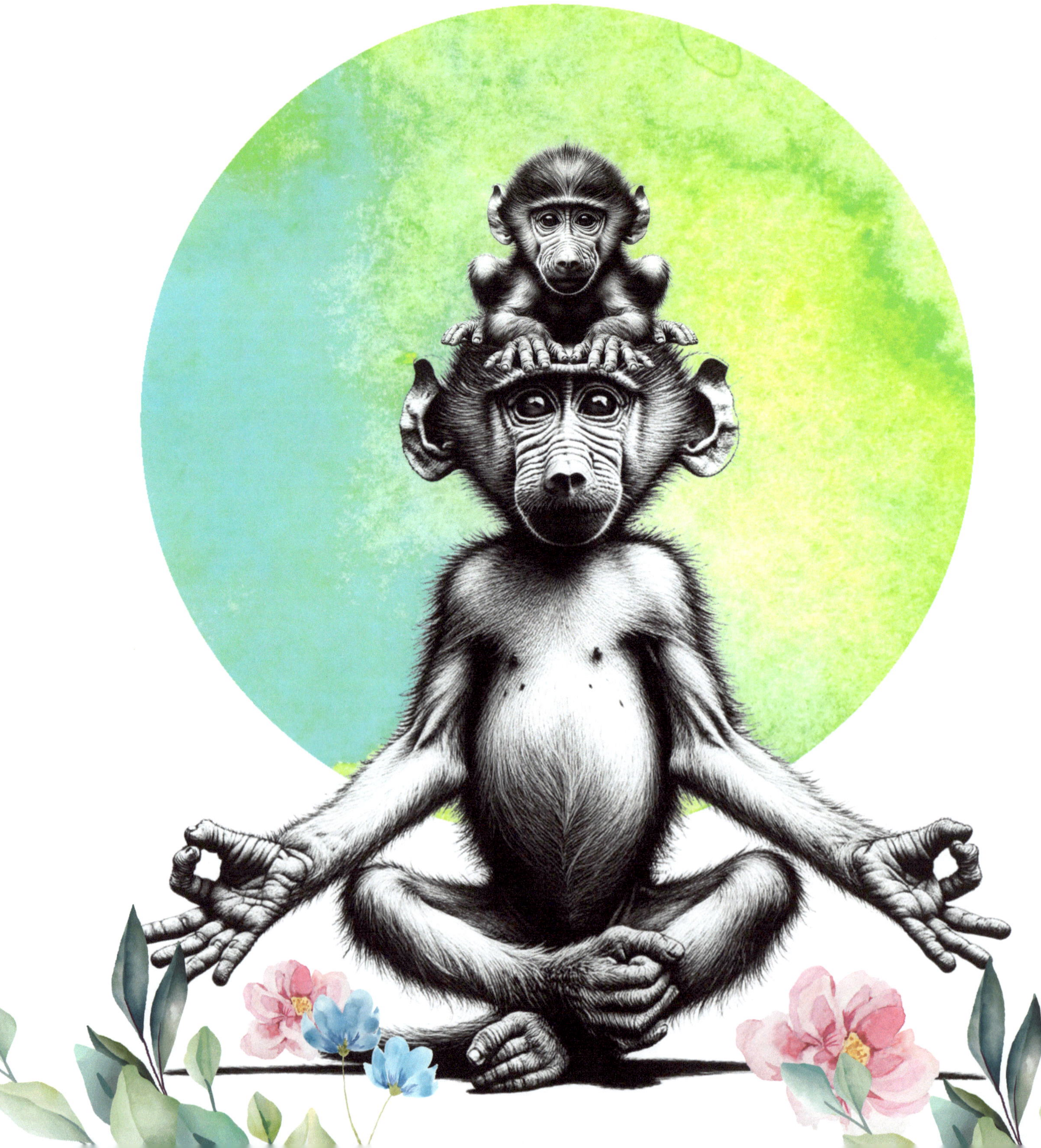

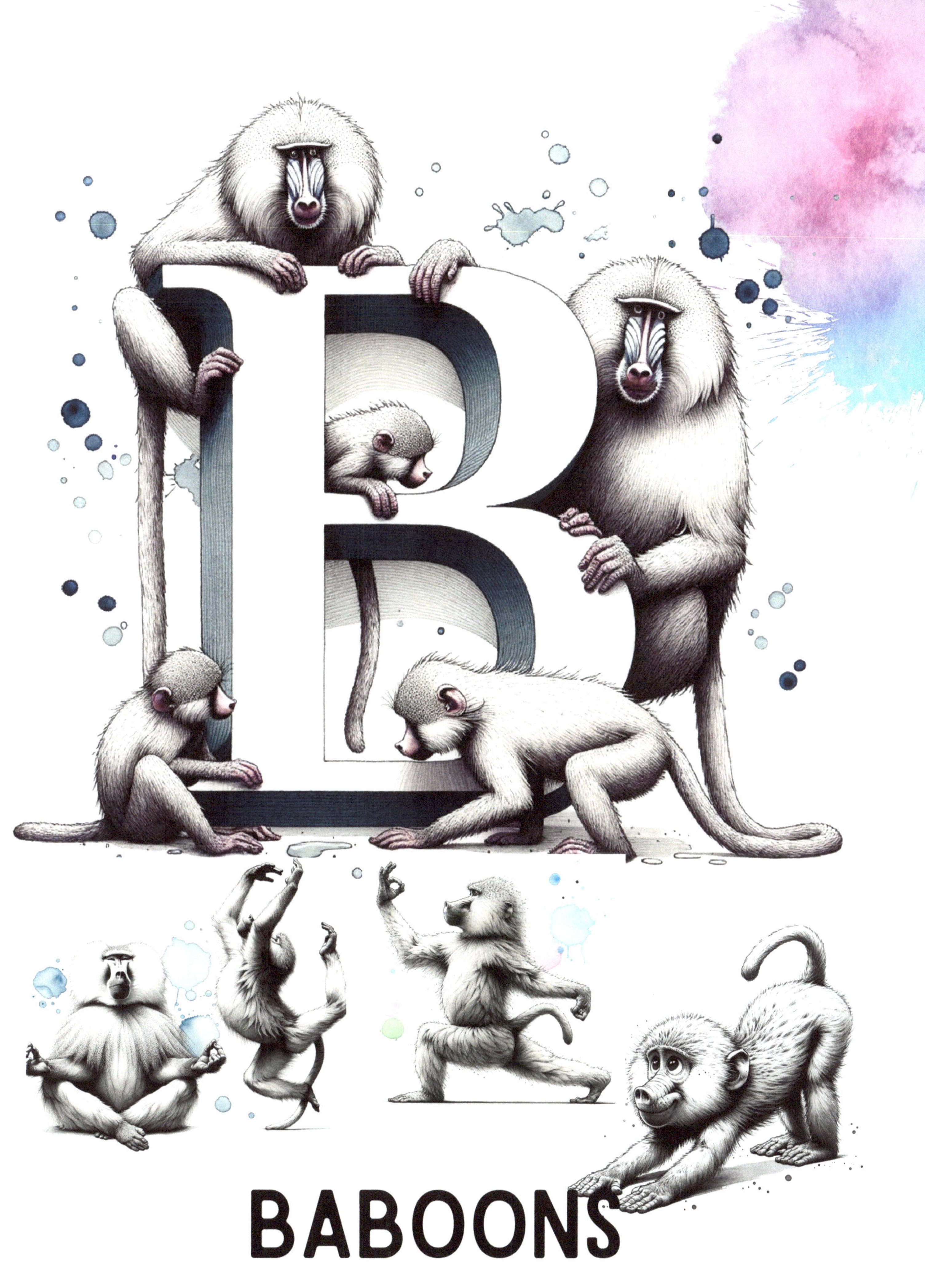

BABOONS

CAPYBARAS ARE THE WORLD'S LARGEST RODENTS. THEY ARE KNOWN FOR BEING EXTREMELY FRIENDLY AND MAKING FRIENDS WITH OTHER ANIMALS.

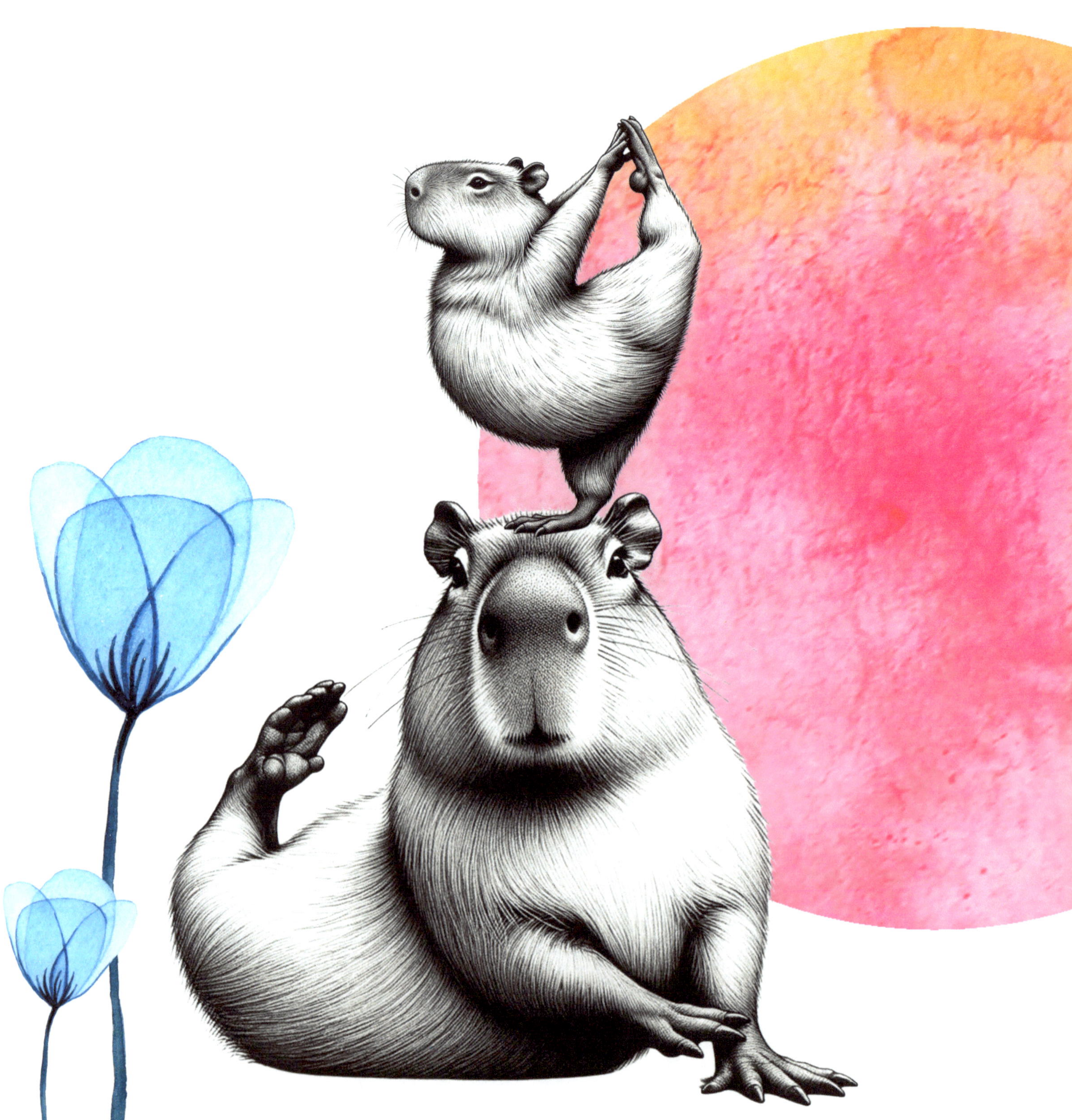

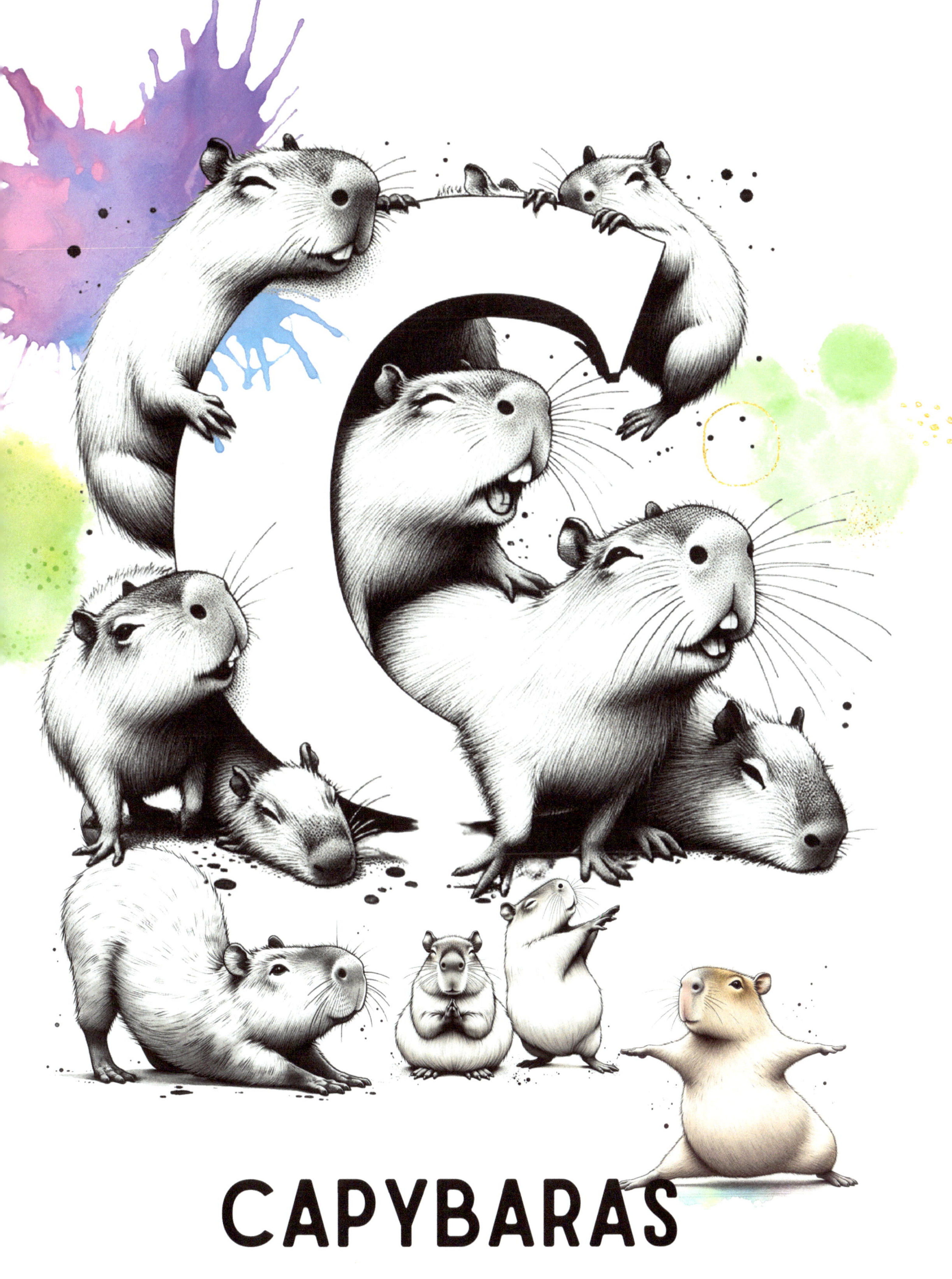

CAPYBARAS

DACHSUND MEANDS "BADGER DOG" IN GERMAN. THEY ARE KNOWN FOR BEING COURAGEOUS AND LOVING, BUT ALSO VERY DIFFICULT TO TRAIN.

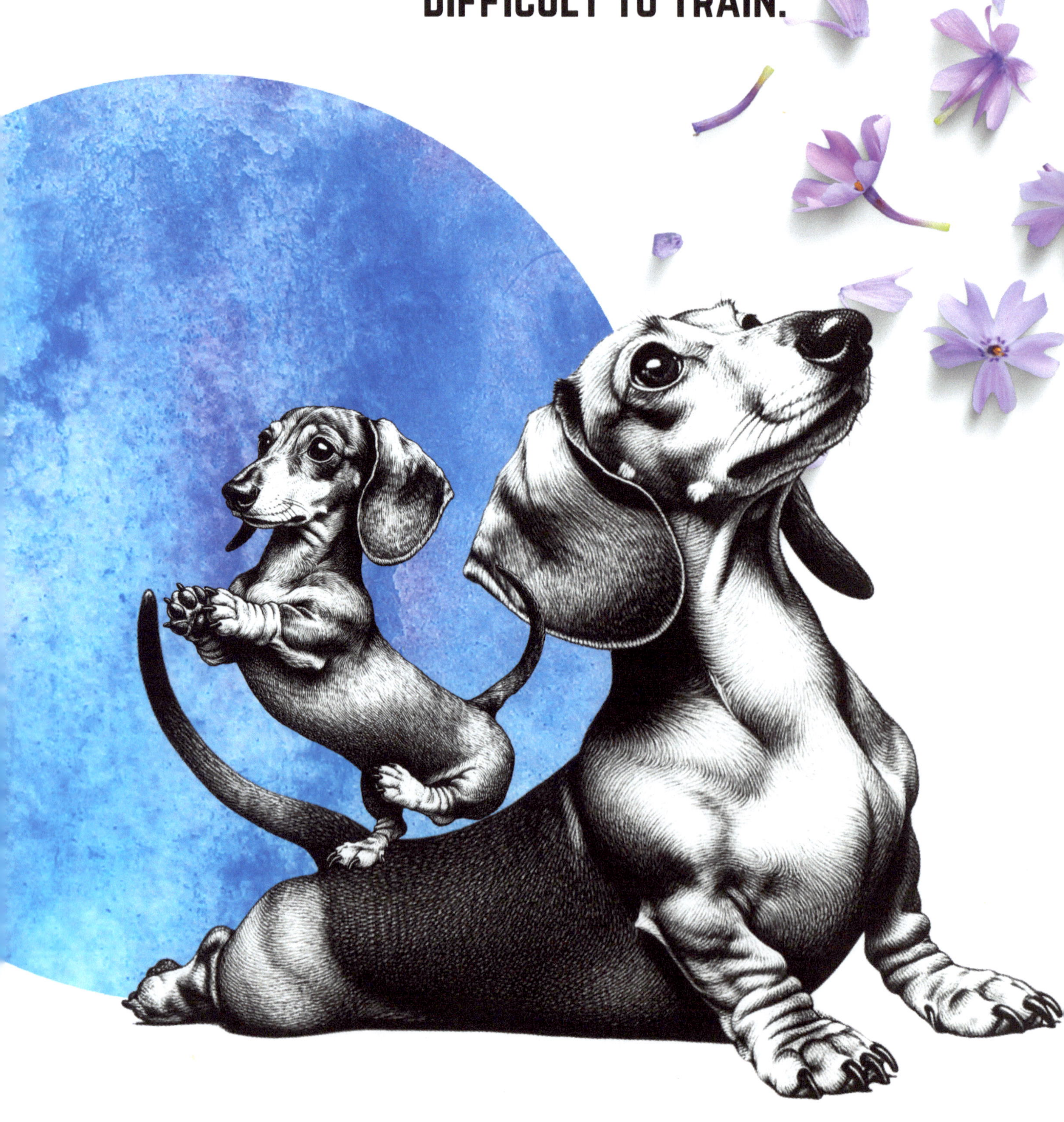

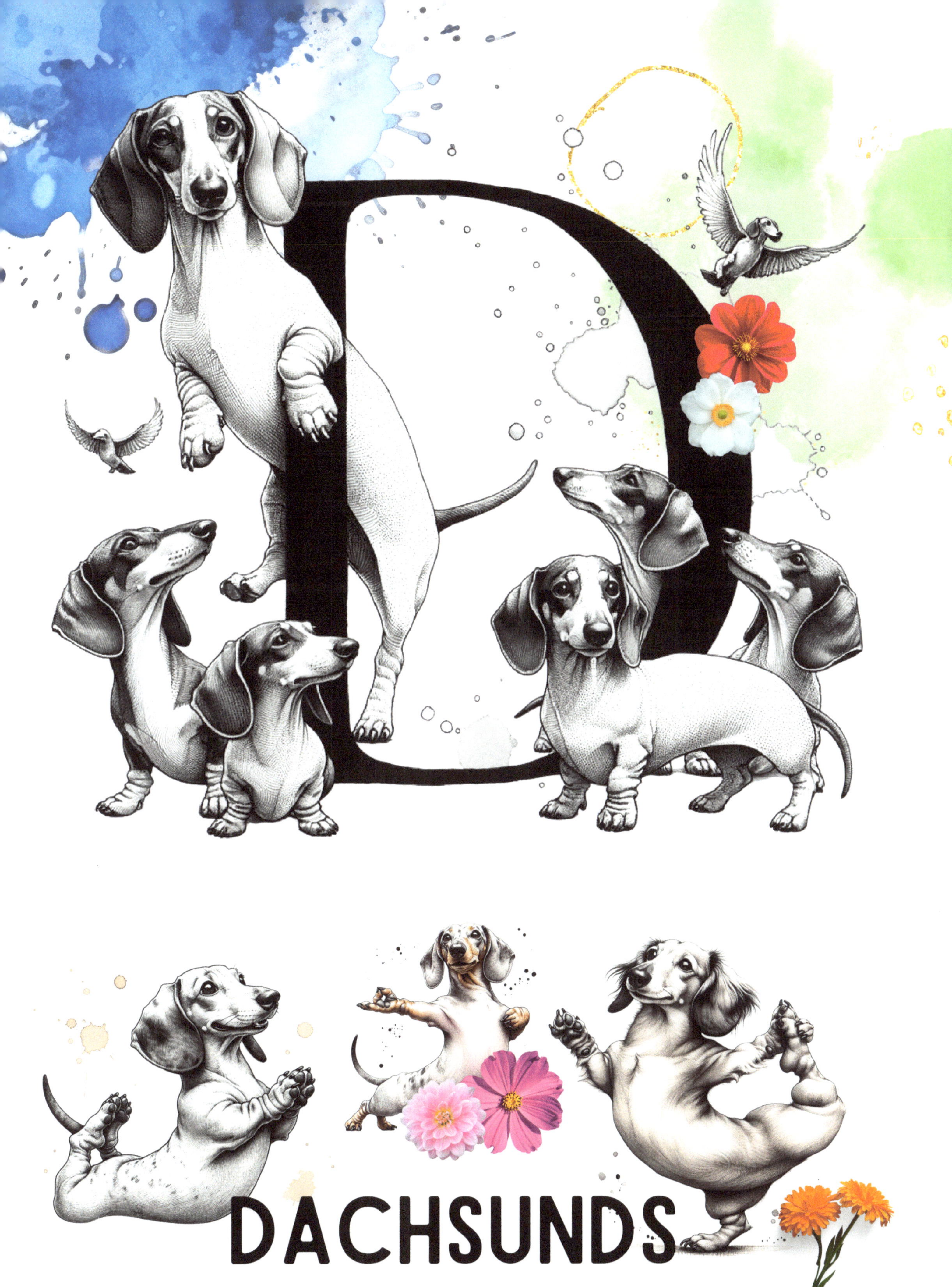

DACHSUNDS

ELEPHANTS ARE THE ONLY MAMMAL THAT CAN'T JUMP. NOT AT ALL. NOT EVEN A LITTLE BIT.

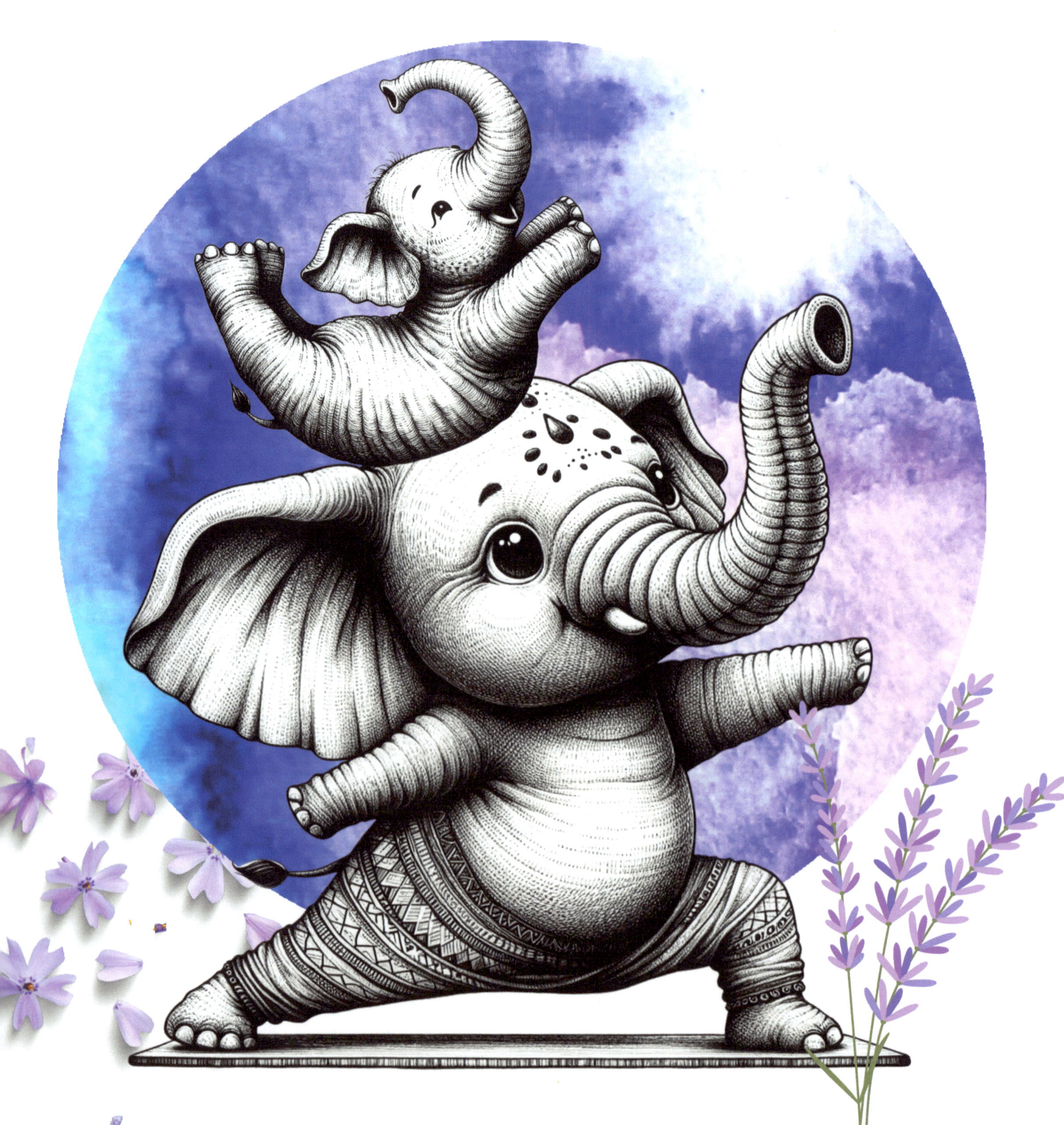

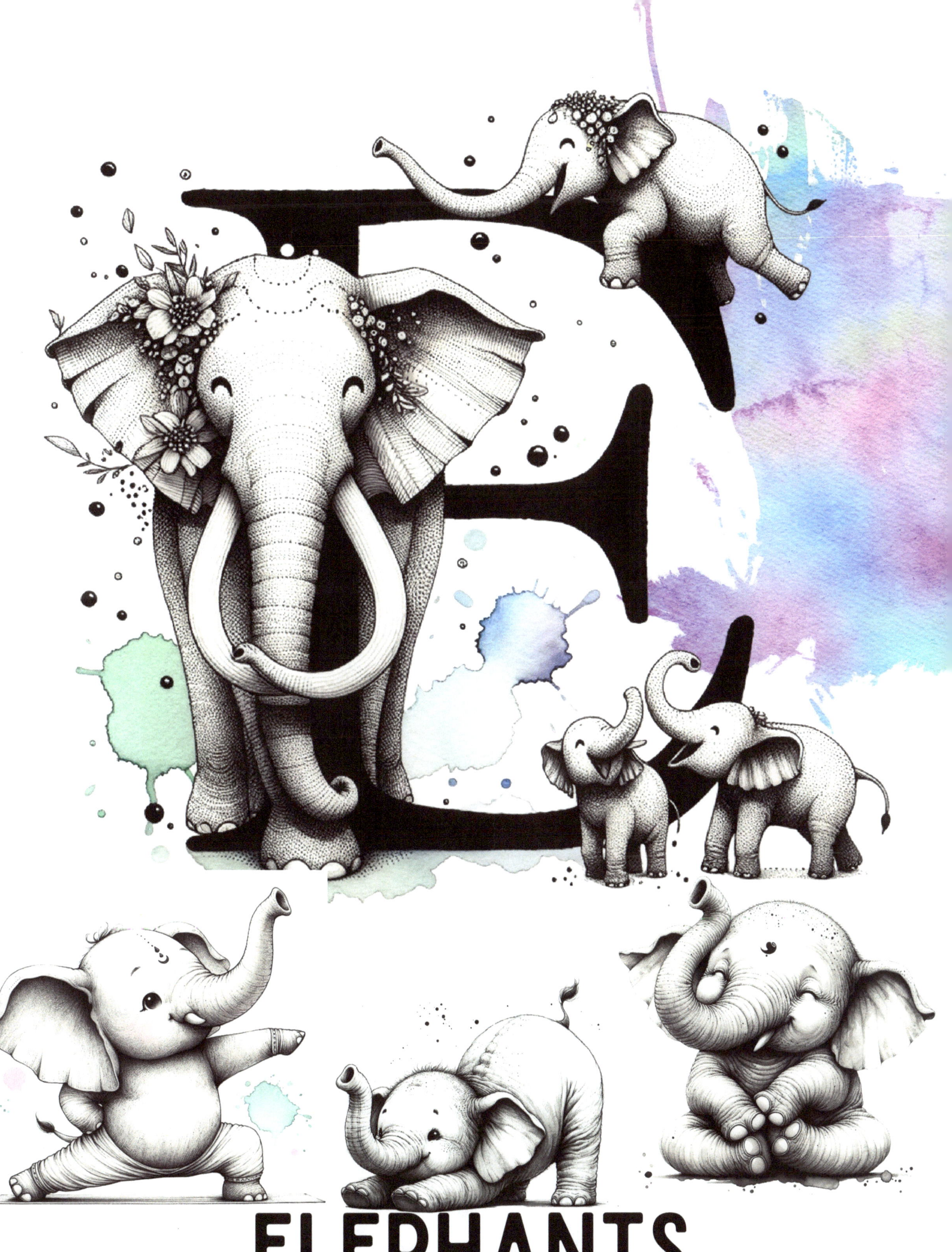

ELEPHANTS

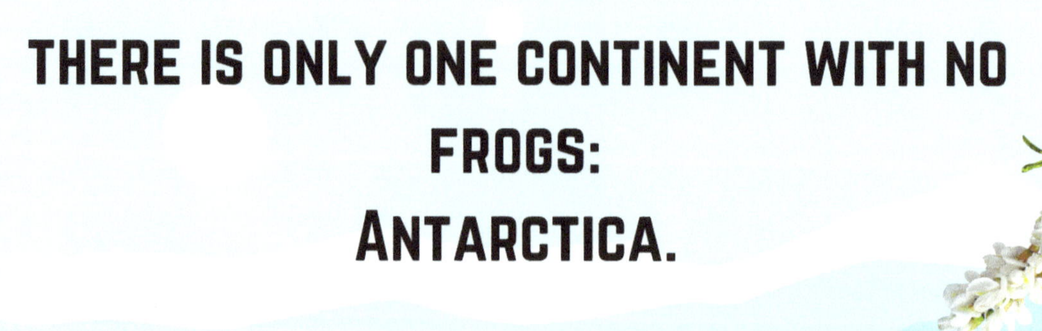
THERE IS ONLY ONE CONTINENT WITH NO FROGS:
ANTARCTICA.

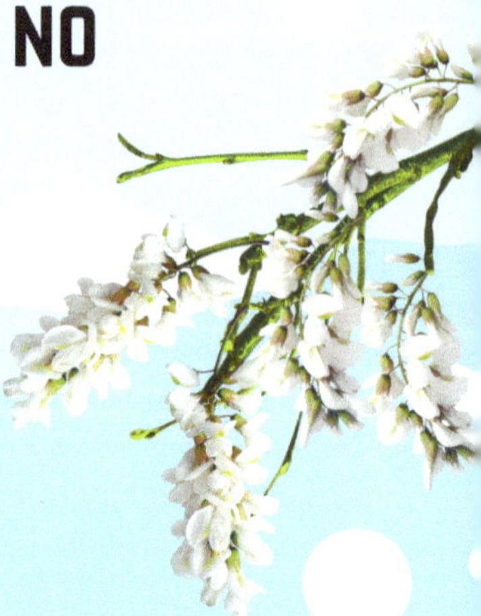

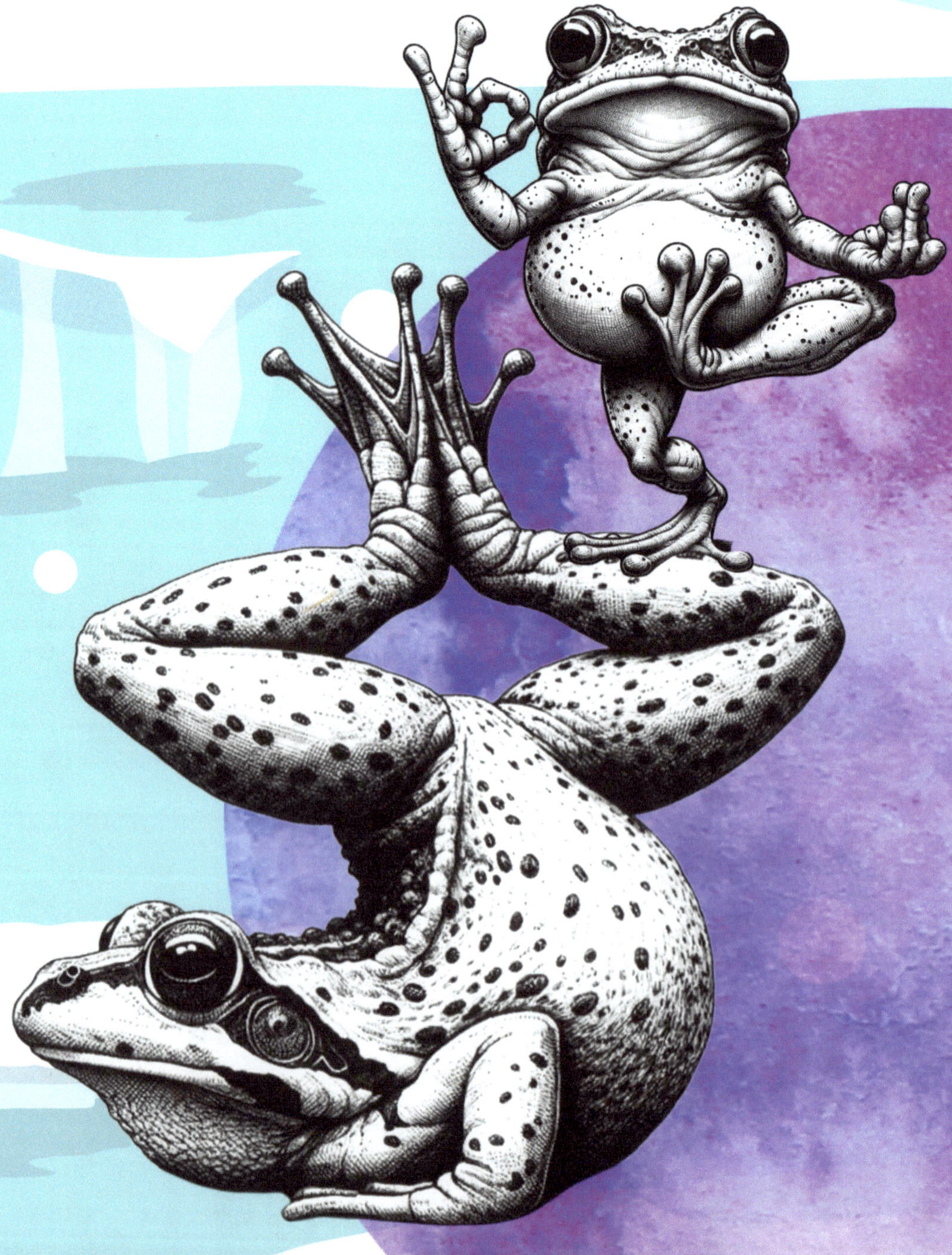

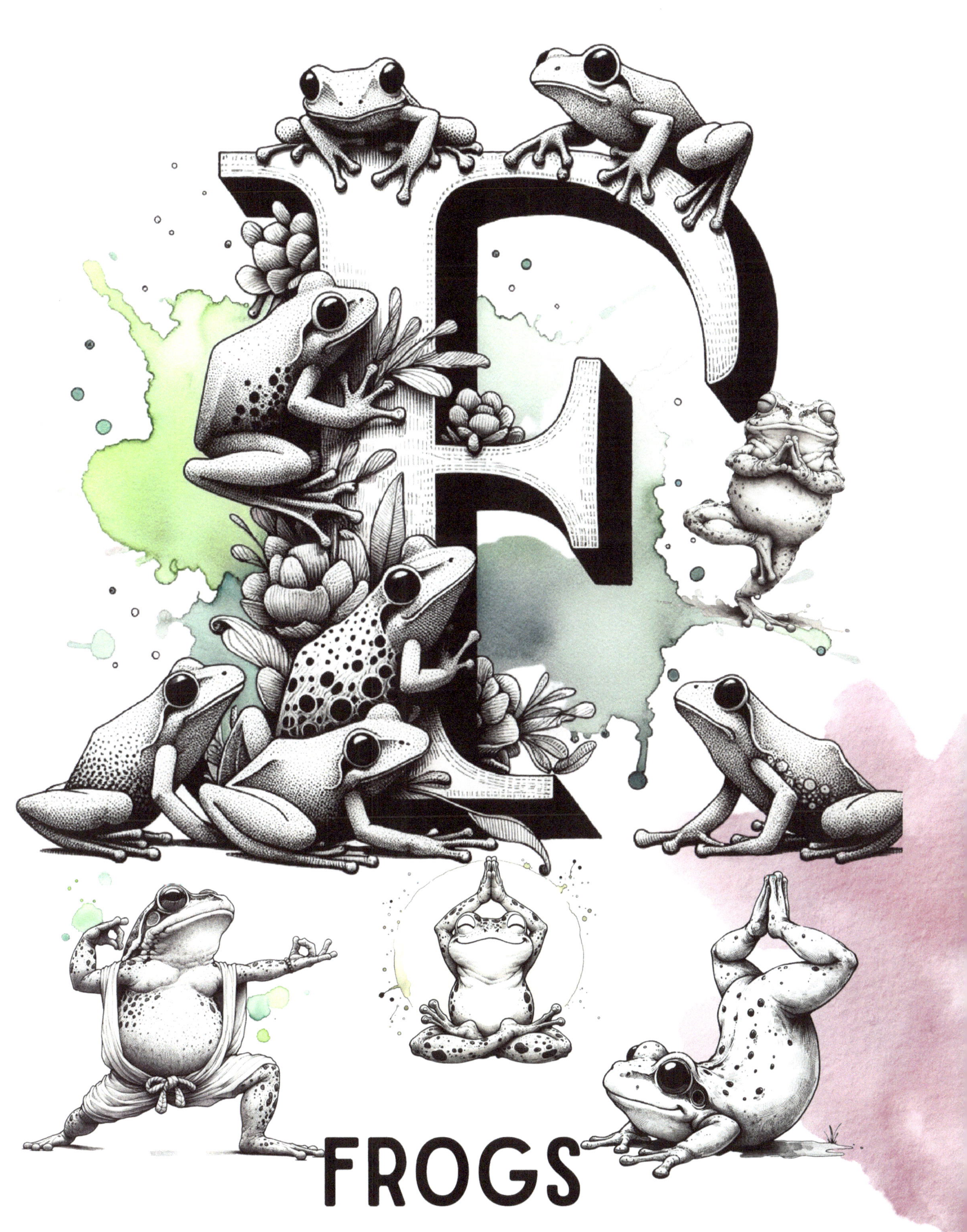

FROGS

JUST THE LEGS OF GIRAFFES ARE TALLER THAN THE AVERAGE HUMAN. THE AVERAGE GIRAFFE IS TALLER THAN THREE ADULT HUMANS.

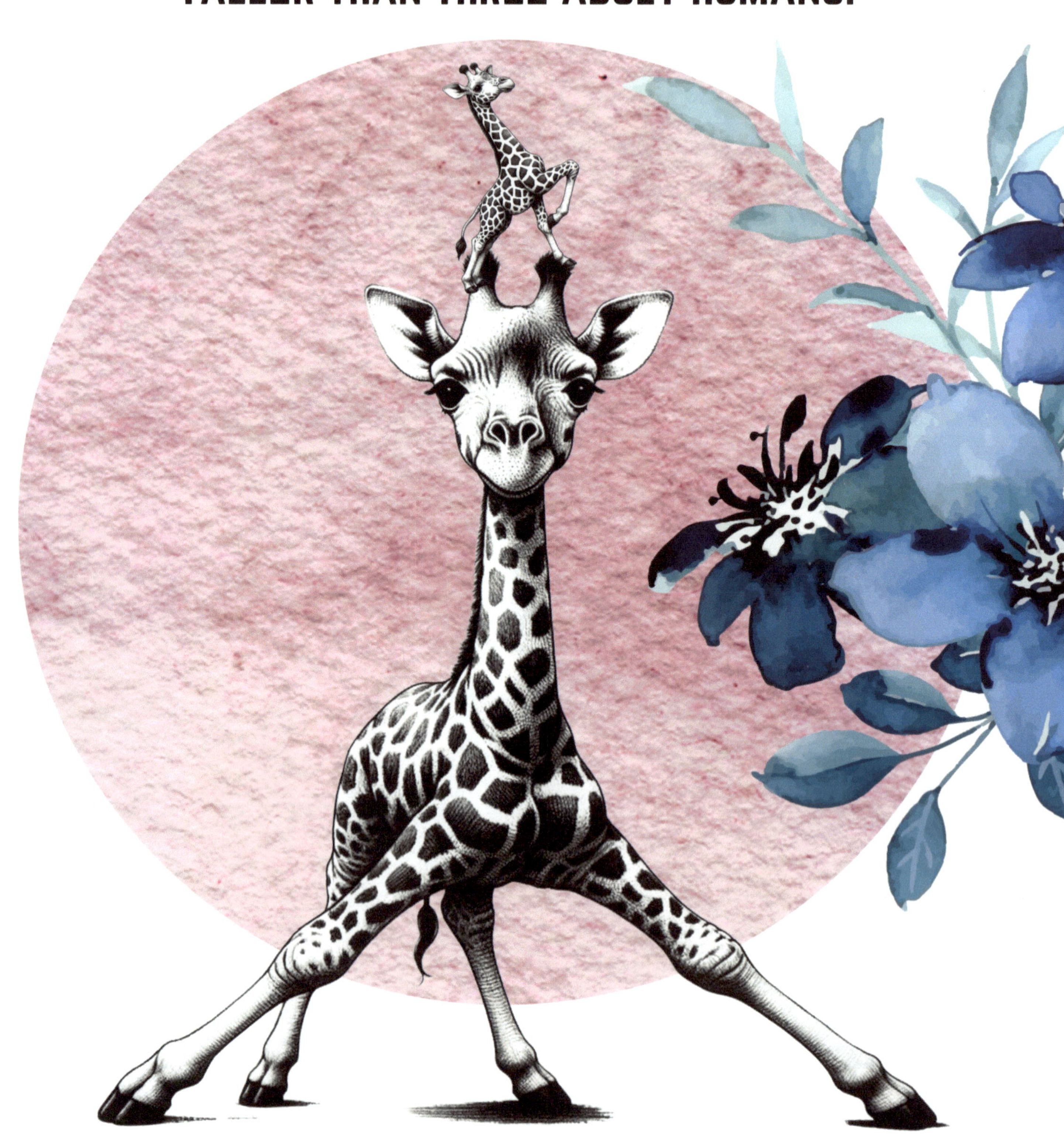

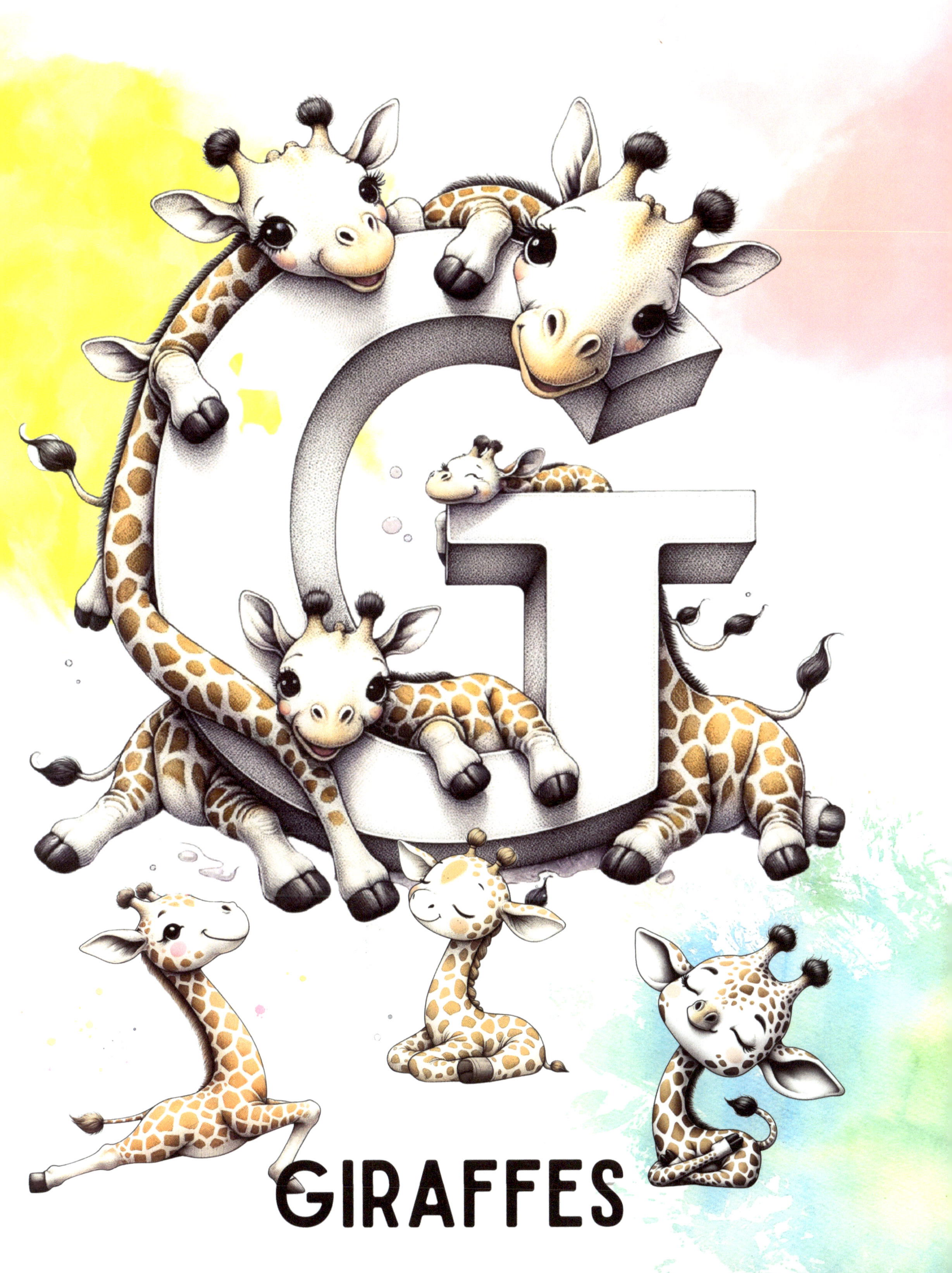

GIRAFFES

HIPPOPOTAMUSES ARE THE SECOND LARGEST LAND ANIMAL ON EARTH. THEY MAY BE CUTE, BUT THEY ARE VERY DANGEROUS AND AGGRESSIVE.

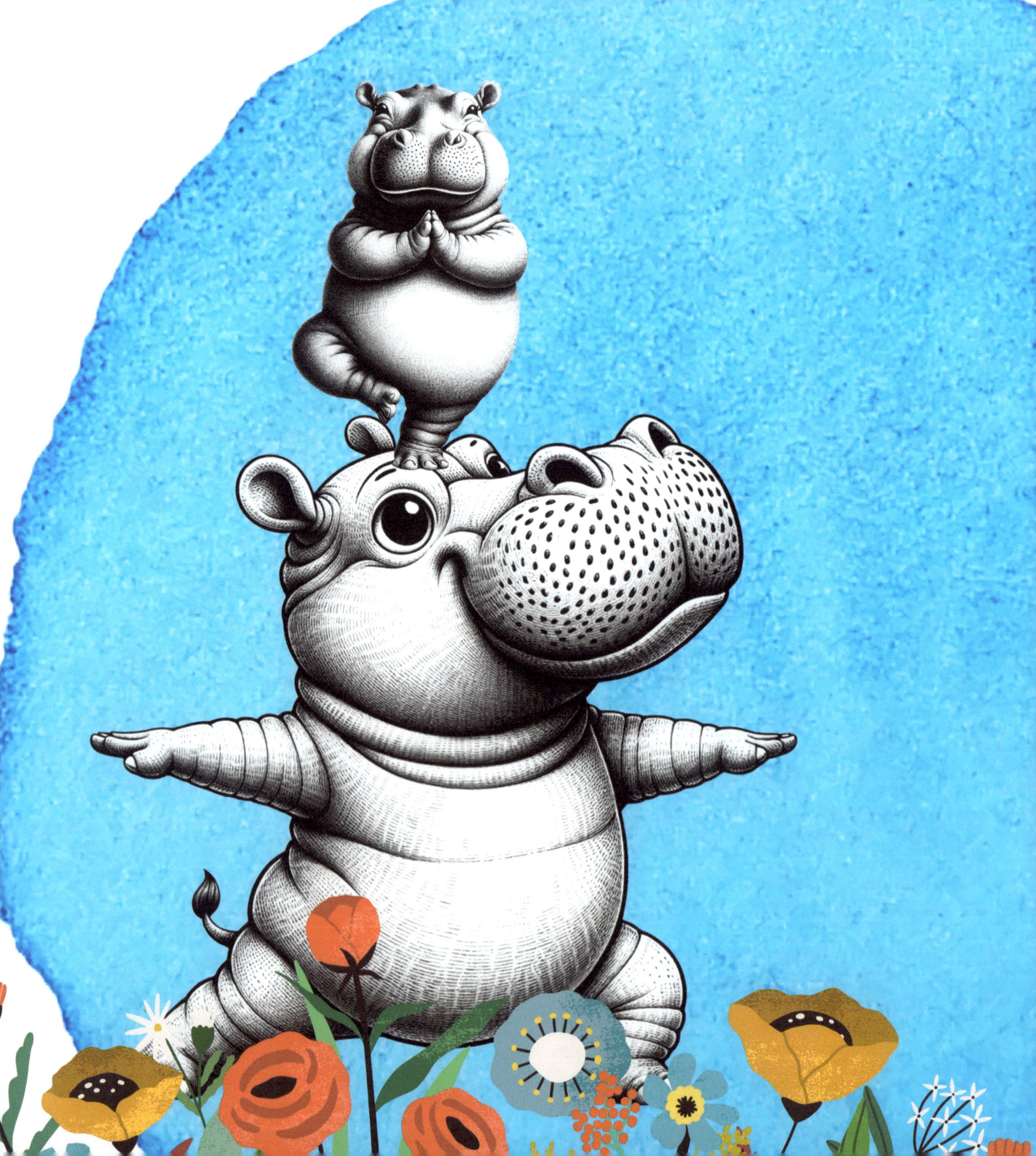

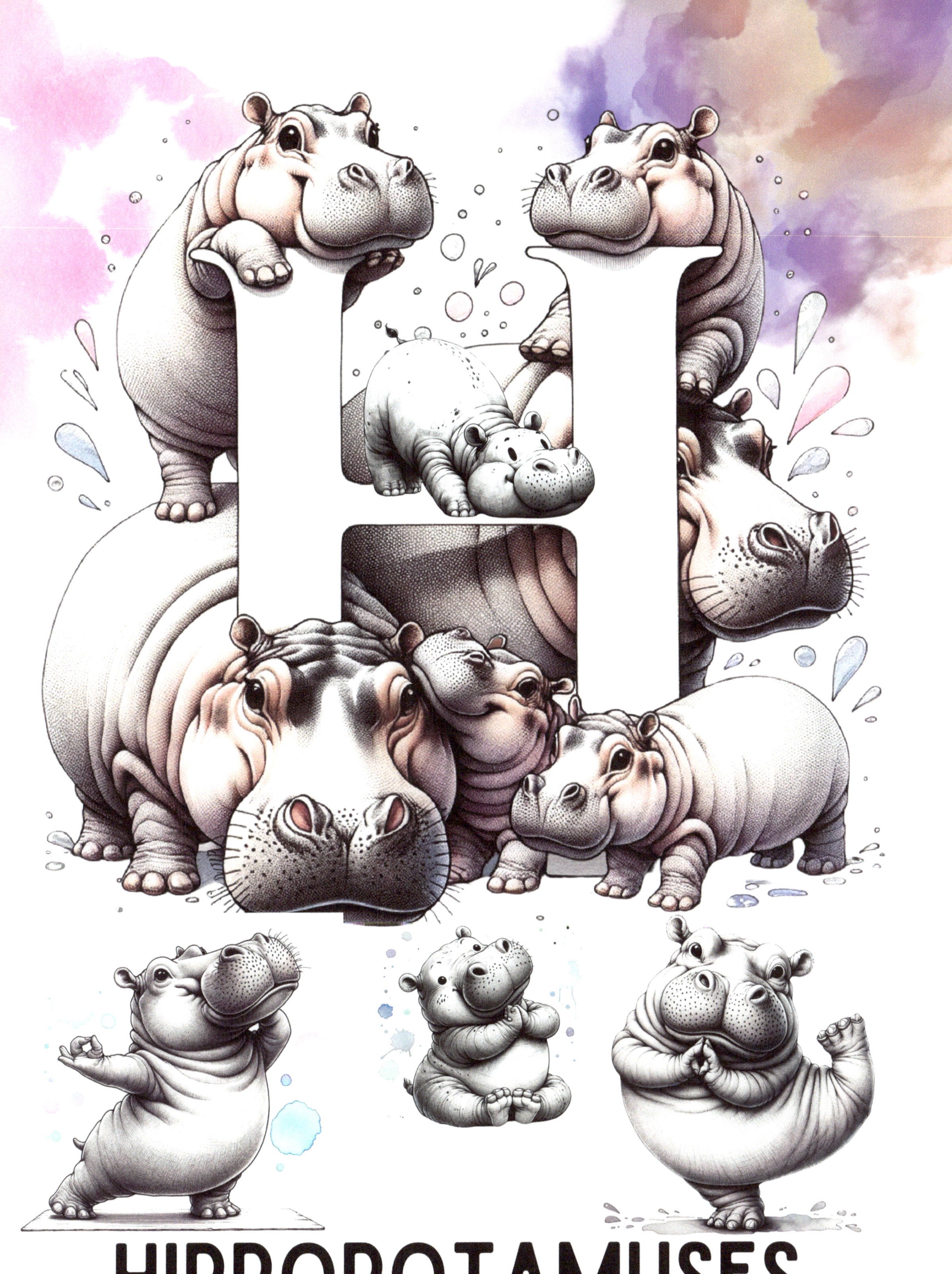

HIPPOPOTAMUSES

IGUANAS ARE AMONG THE LARGEST LIZARDS IN THE WORLD. THEY CAN GROW UP TO SIX AND A HALF FEET LONG. THEY CAN ALSO SEE IN COLOR.

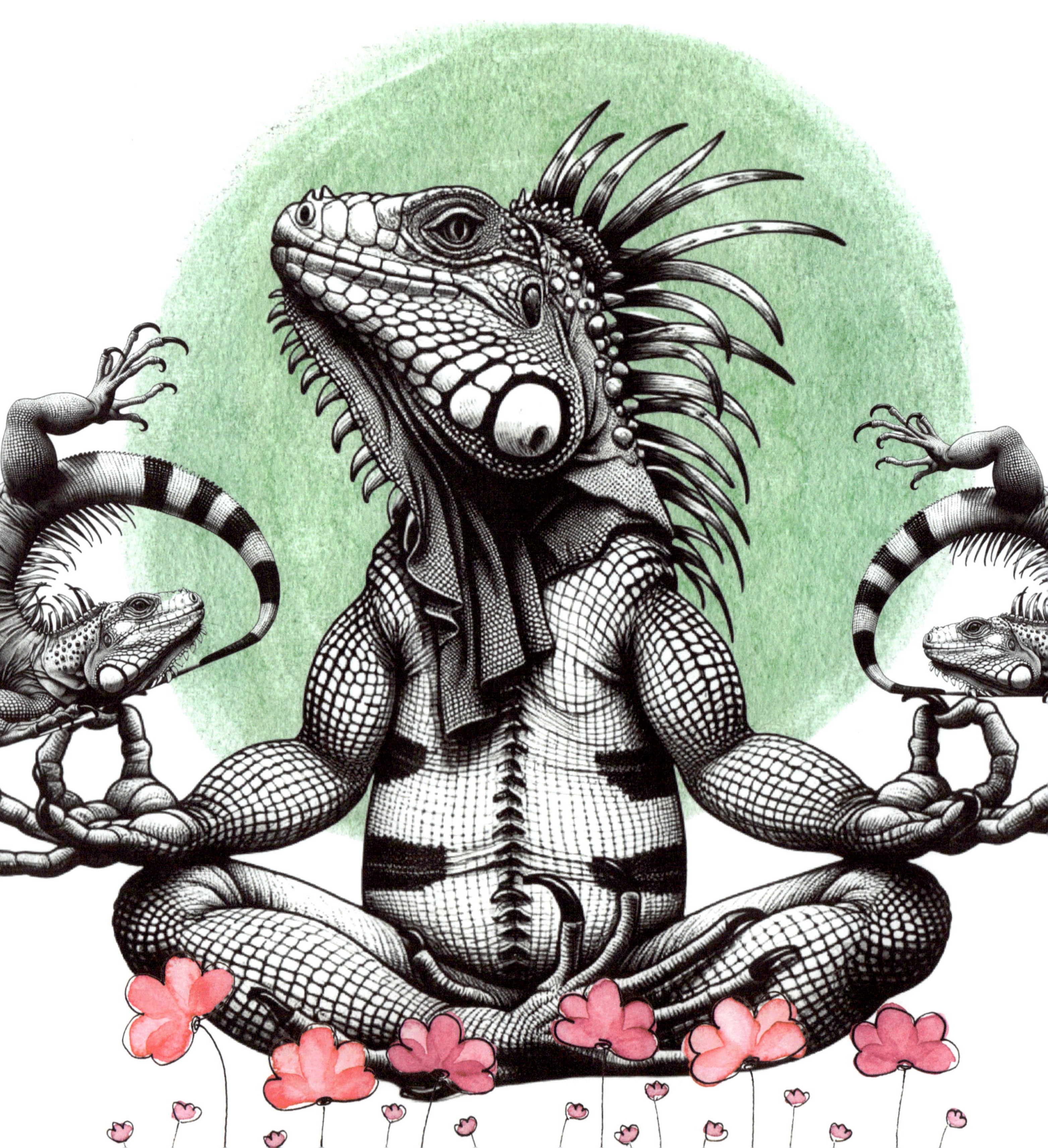

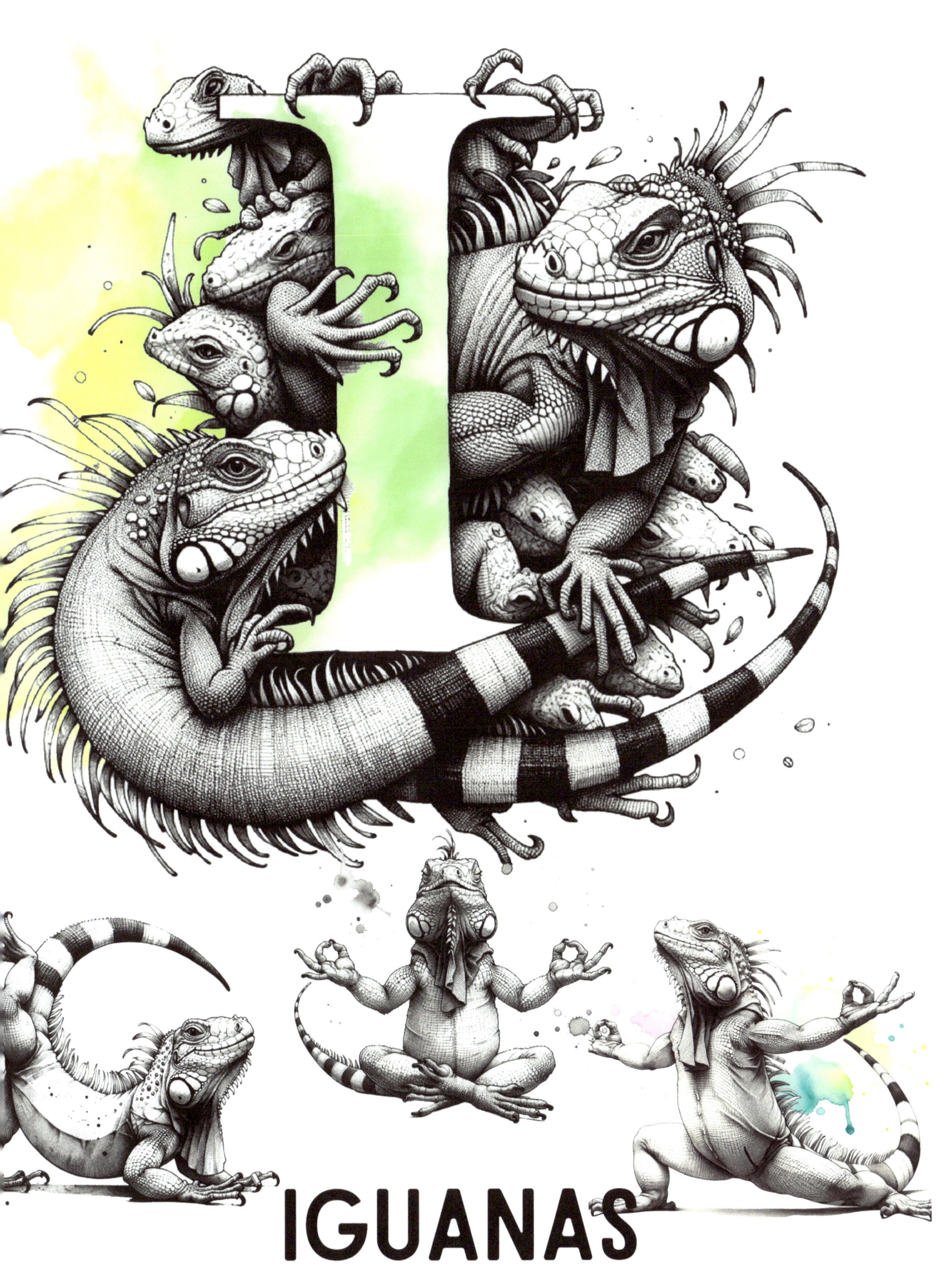
IGUANAS

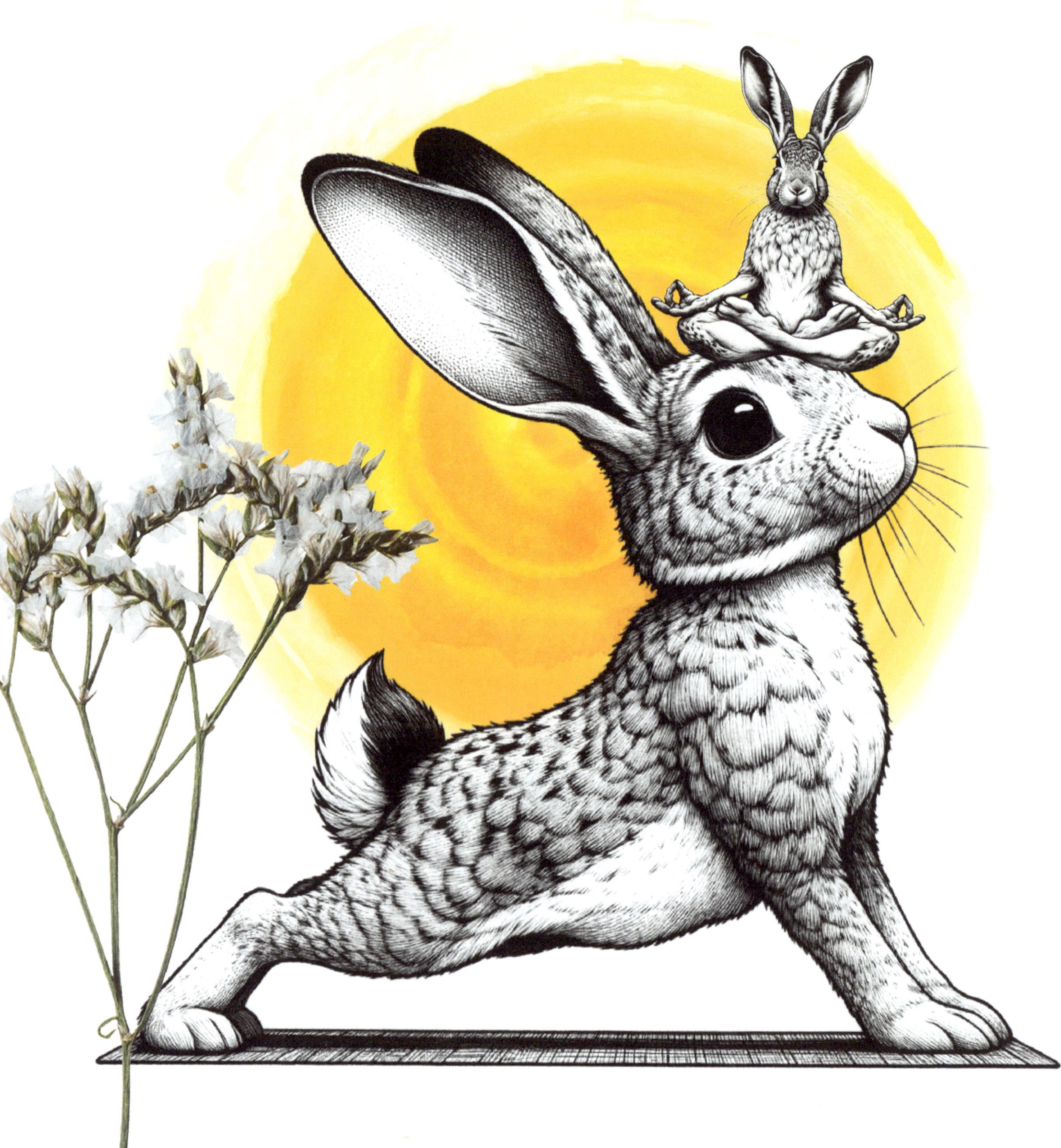

JACKRABBITS ARE ACTUALLY NOT RABBITS, THEY ARE HARES. THEIR BABIES ARE BORN WITH THEIR EYES WIDE OPEN.

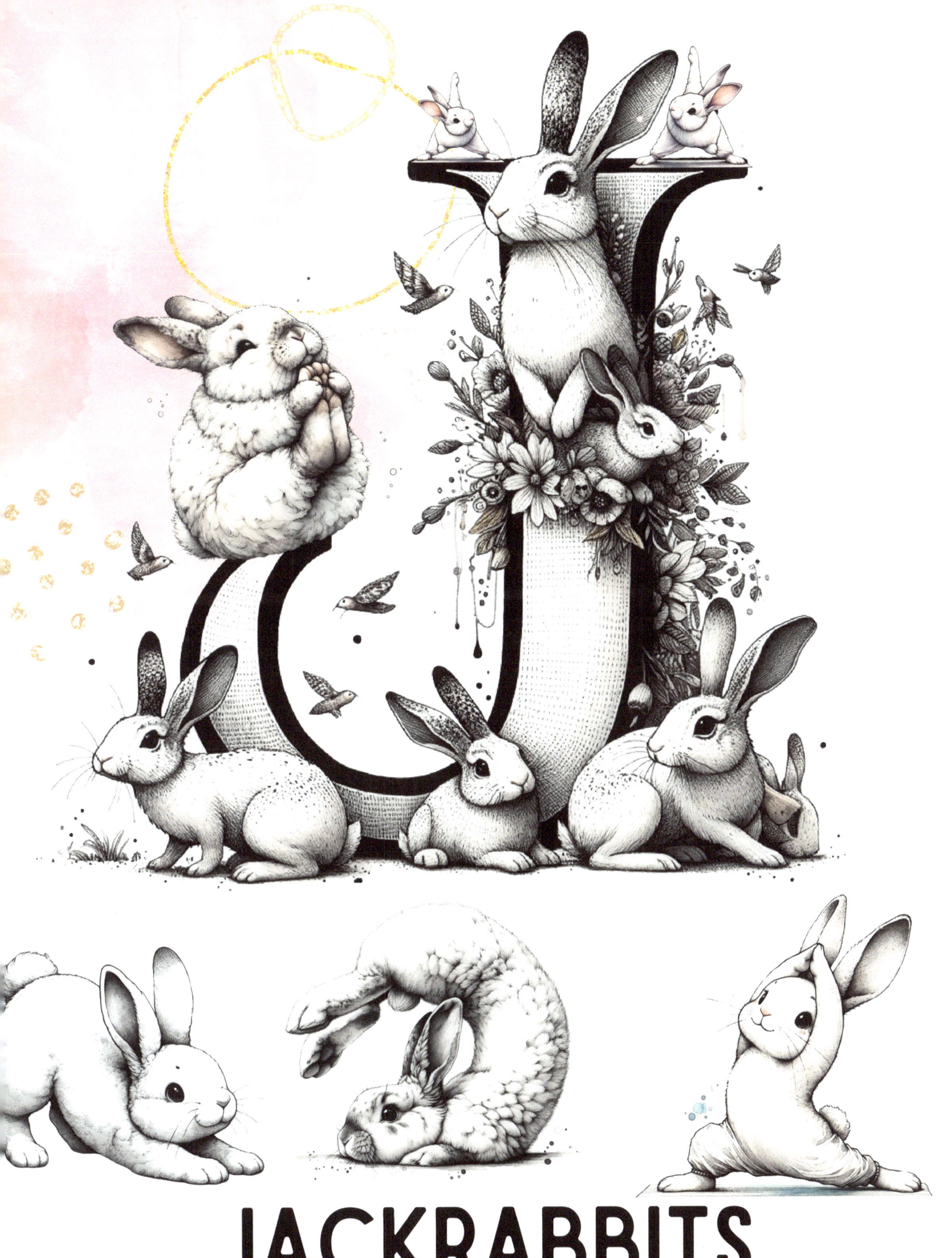

JACKRABBITS

Kangaroos are mostly nocturnal, so they sleep during the day and enjoy the night life. They live an average of six years in the wild.

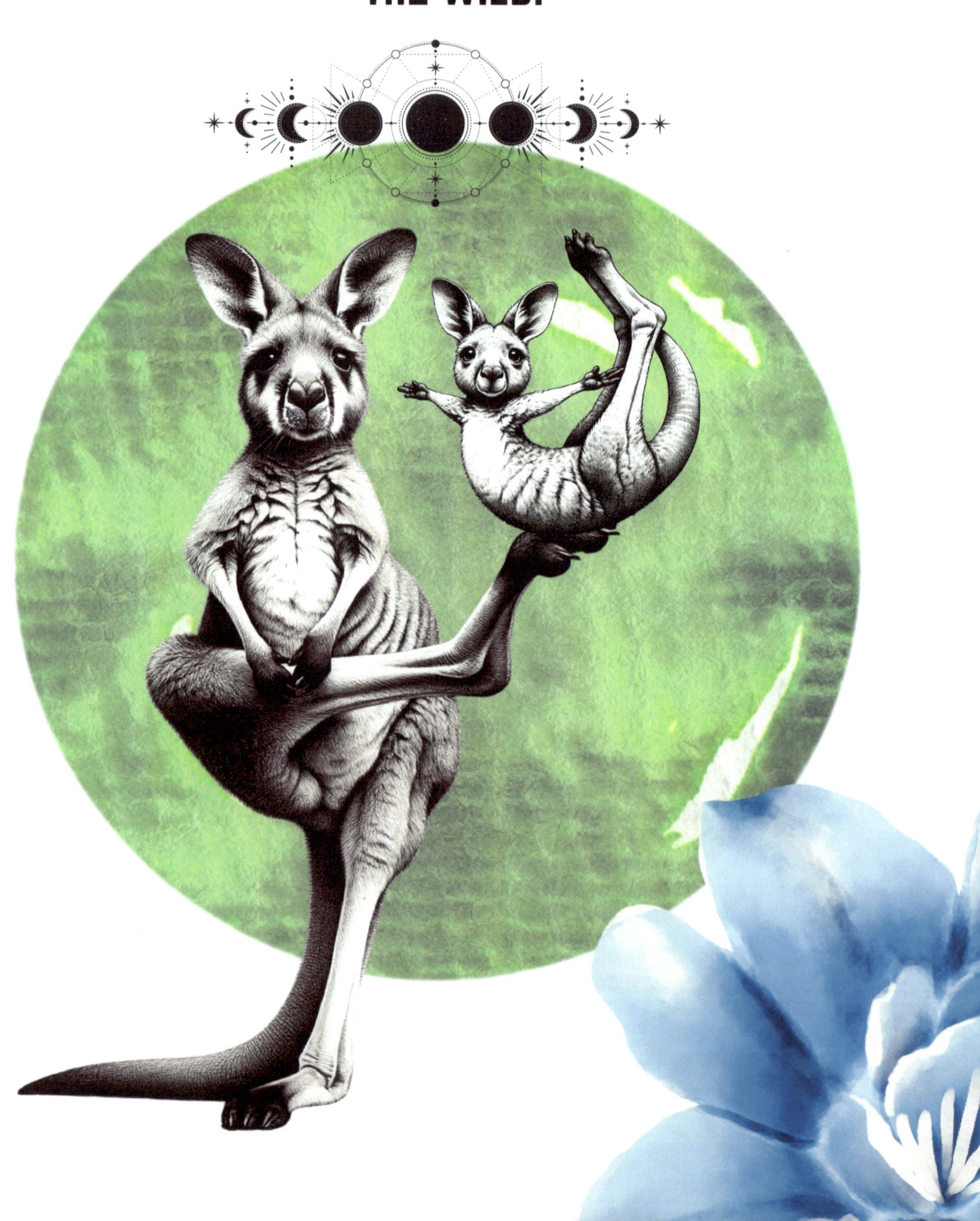

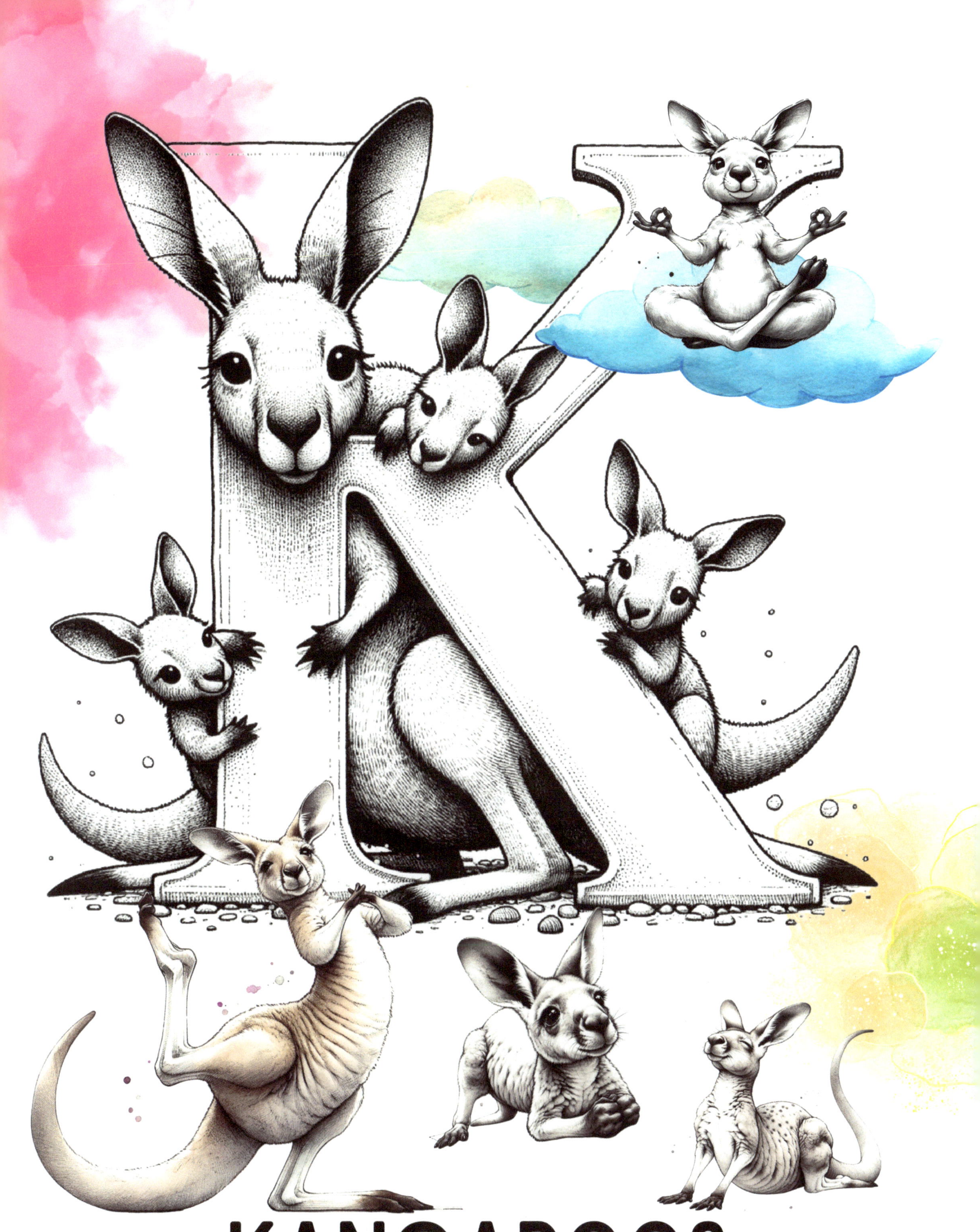

KANGAROOS

LIONS ARE KNOWN AS "APEX PREDATORS". THIS MEAN THEY HAVE NO NATURAL PREDATORS OF THEIR OWN. THIS IS WHY THEY'RE OFTEN CALLED "KING OF THE ANIMALS"

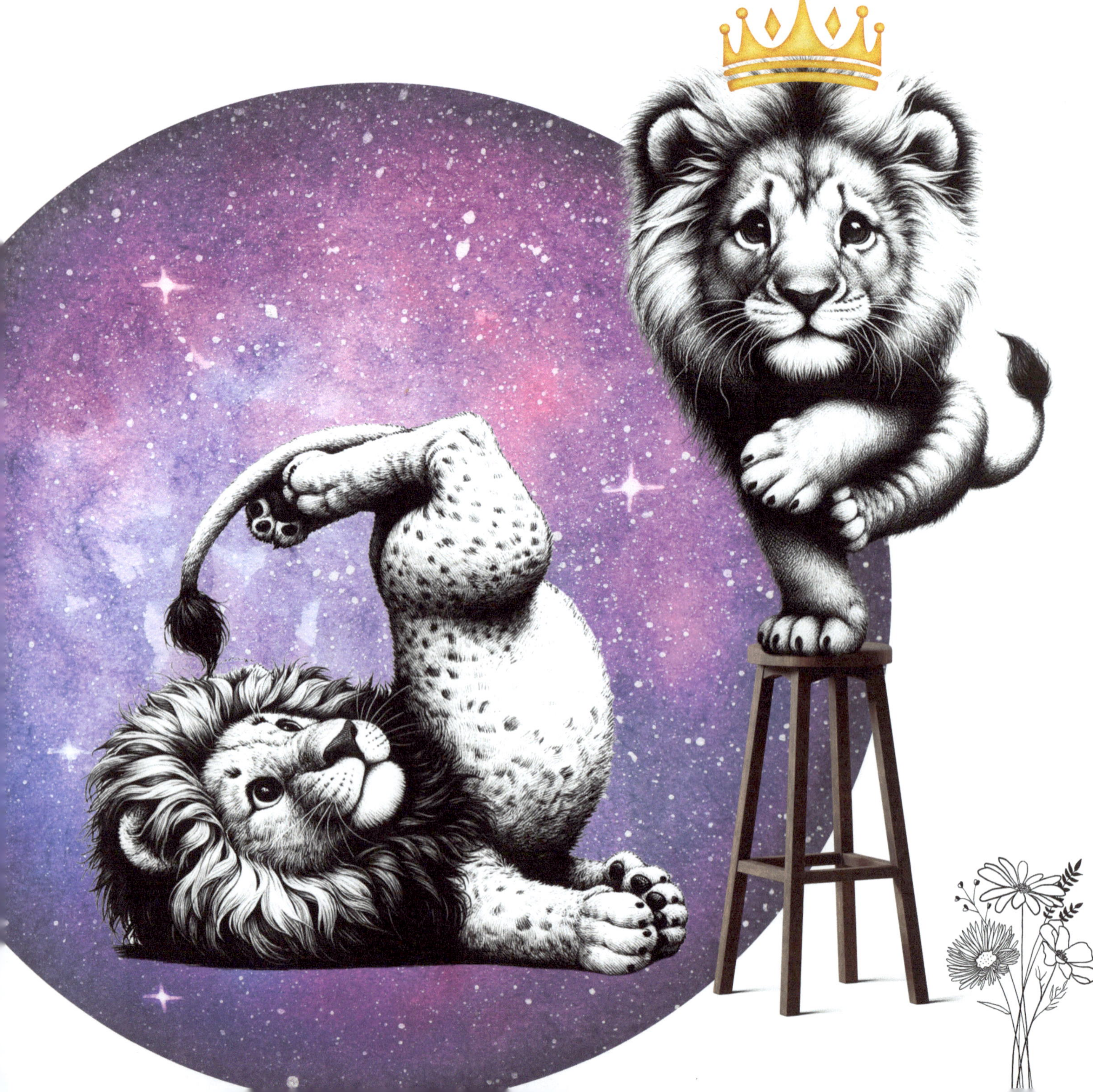

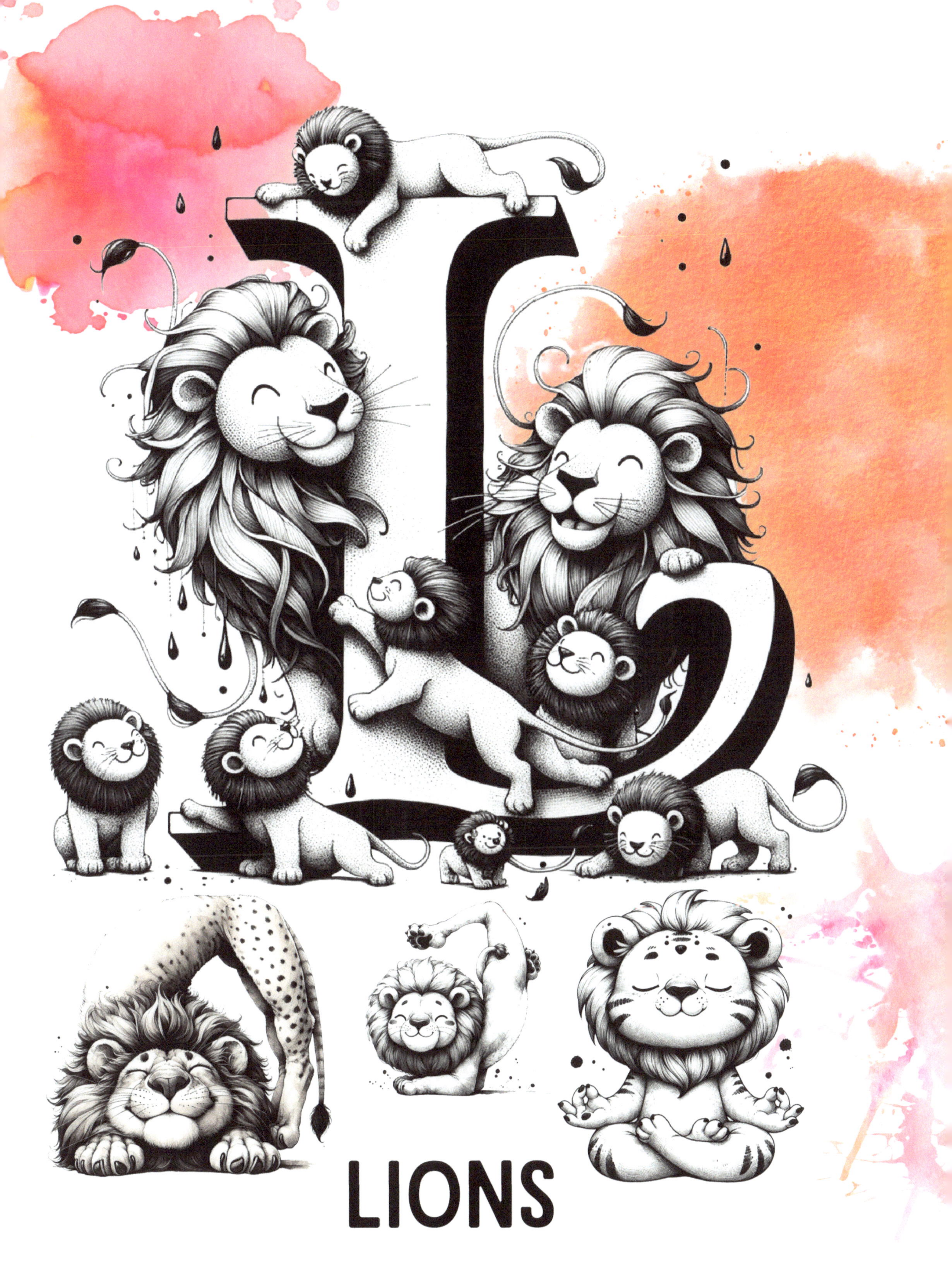

LIONS

MANATEES SPEND HALF THEIR TIME SLEEPING UNDERWATER. THEY COME UP FOR AIR ABOUT EVERY 5 MINUTES. THEY ARE KNOWN FOR BEING VERY SLOW SWIMMERS.

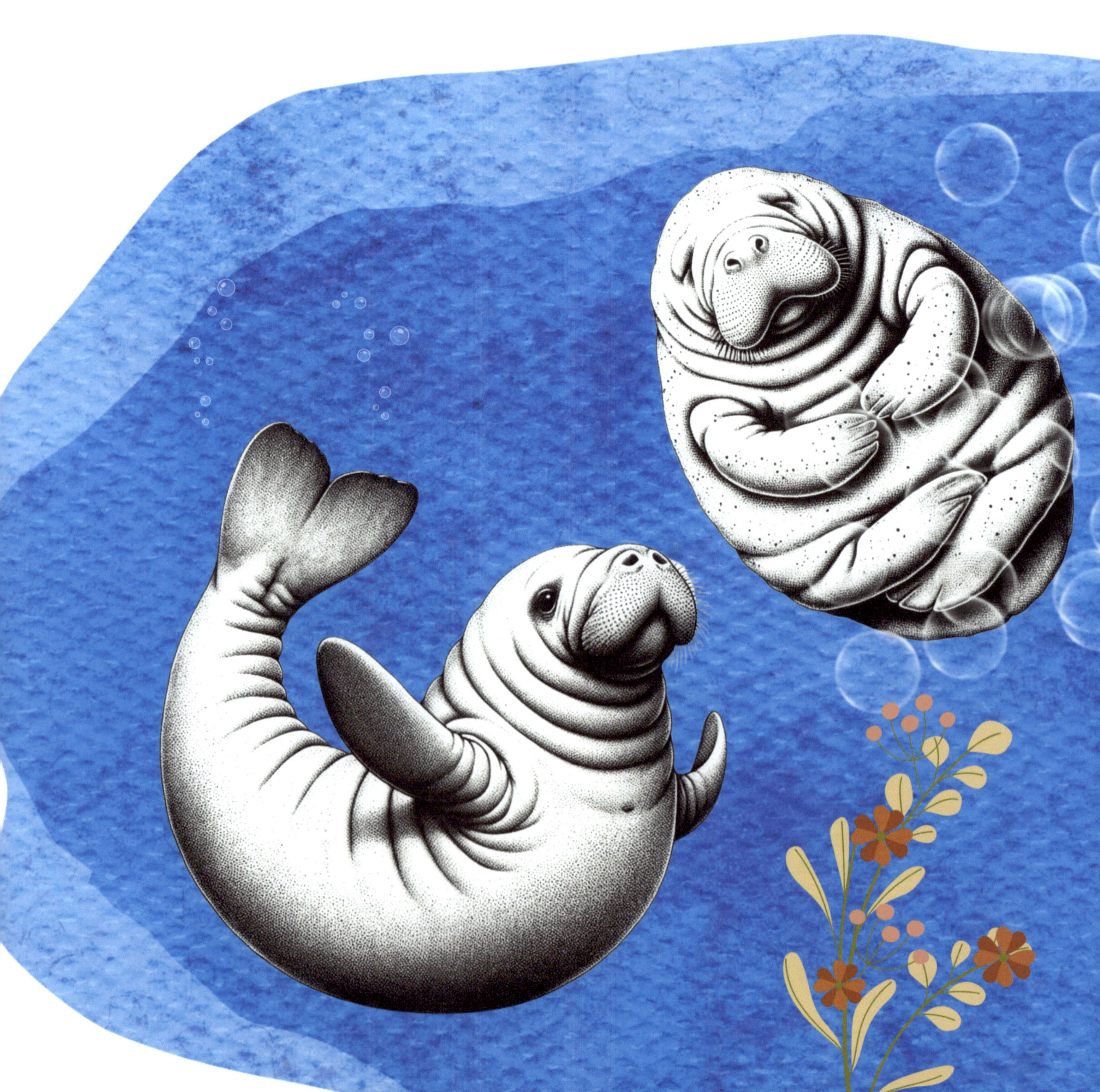

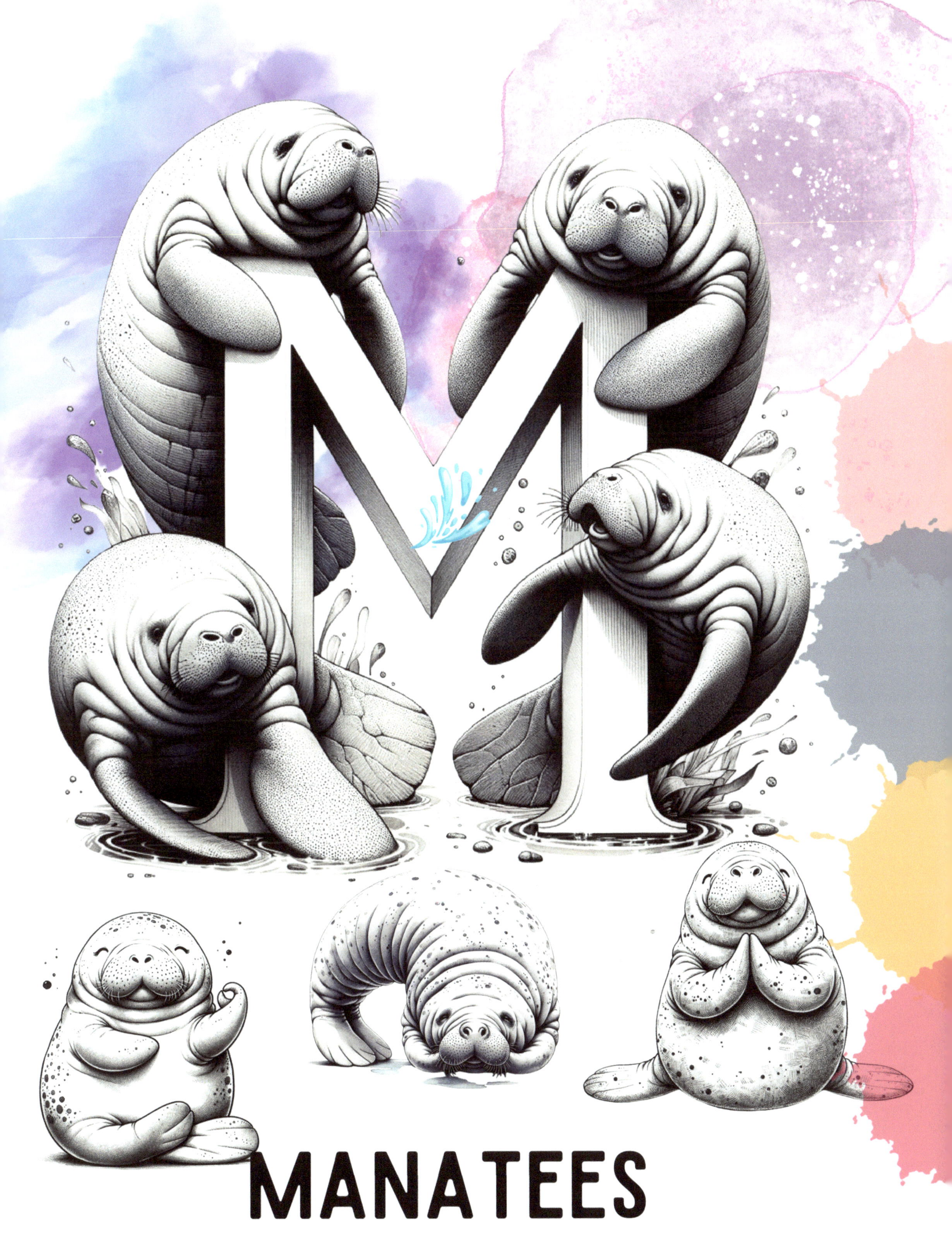

MANATEES

NARWHALS ARE OFTEN CALLED "UNICORNS OF THE SEA" BECAUSE OF THEIR LONG, SPIRAL SHAPED TUSK THAT GROWS FROM THEIR JAW. HOWEVER, ONLY MALE NARWHALS HAVE A TUSK.

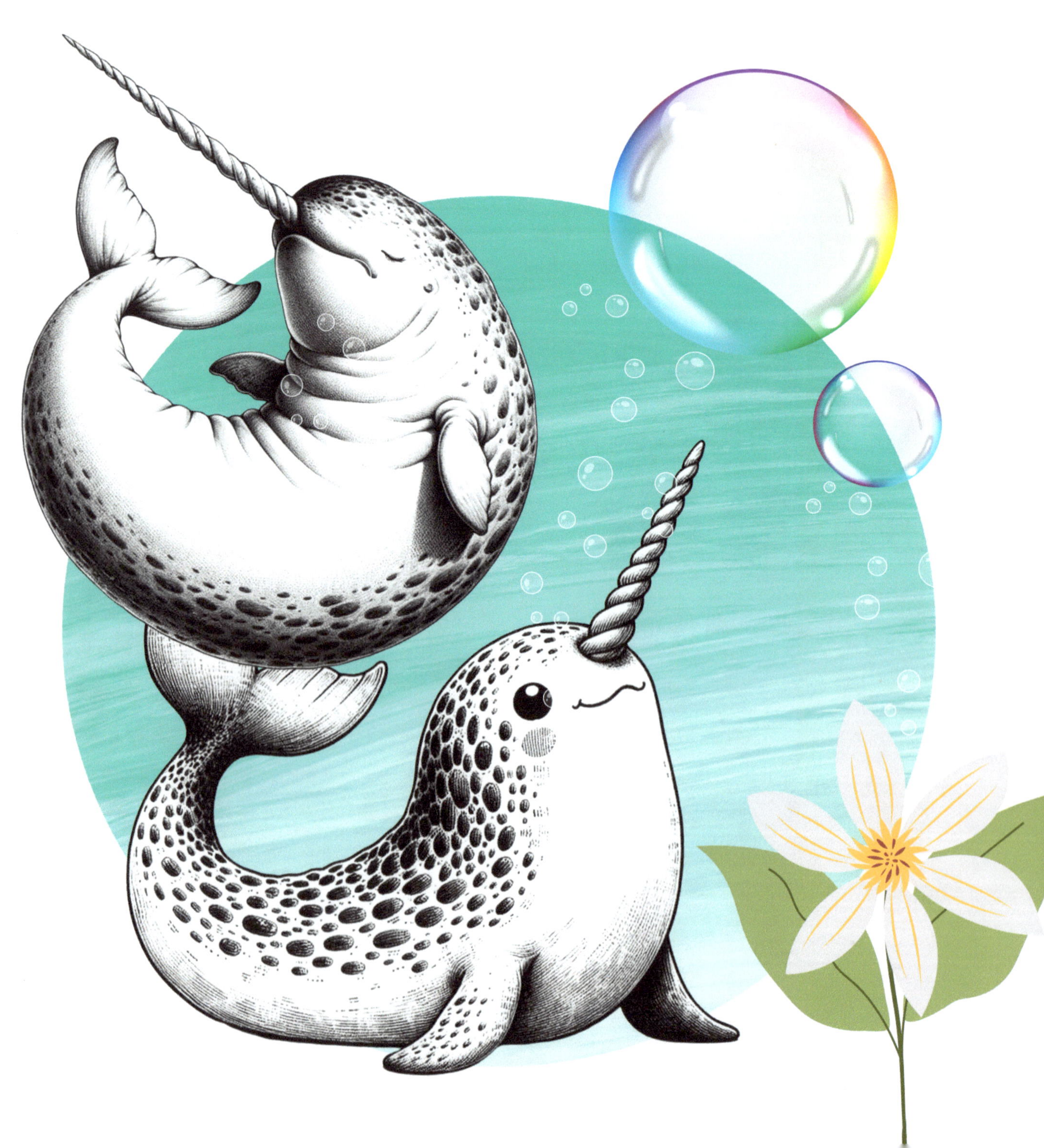

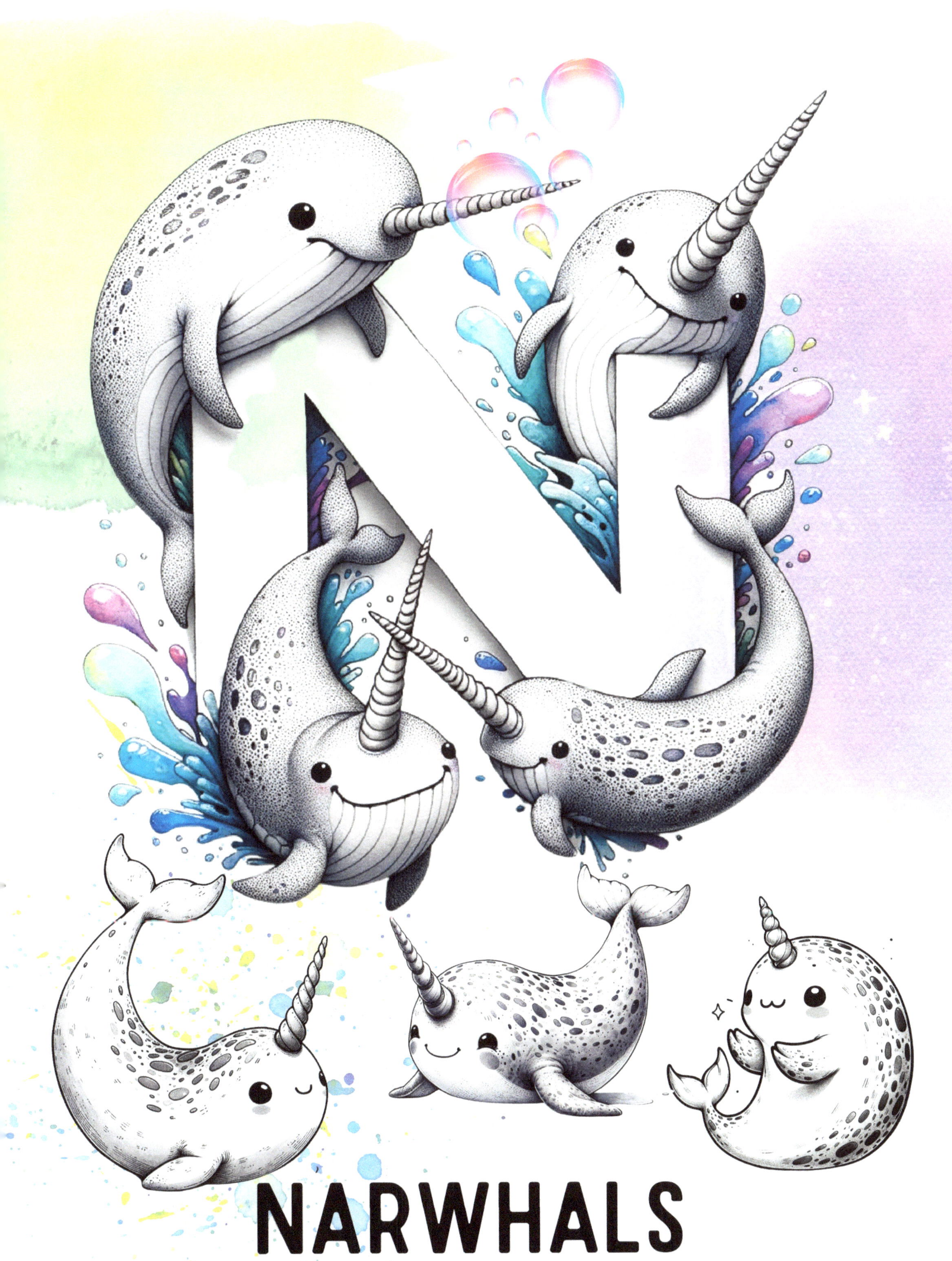

NARWHALS

OTTERS ARE SO GOOD AT FLOATING ON THEIR BACKS. THIS IS BECAUSE THEIR THICK FUR ACTUALLY TRAPS AIR AND HELPS THEM STAY ON THE SURFACE.

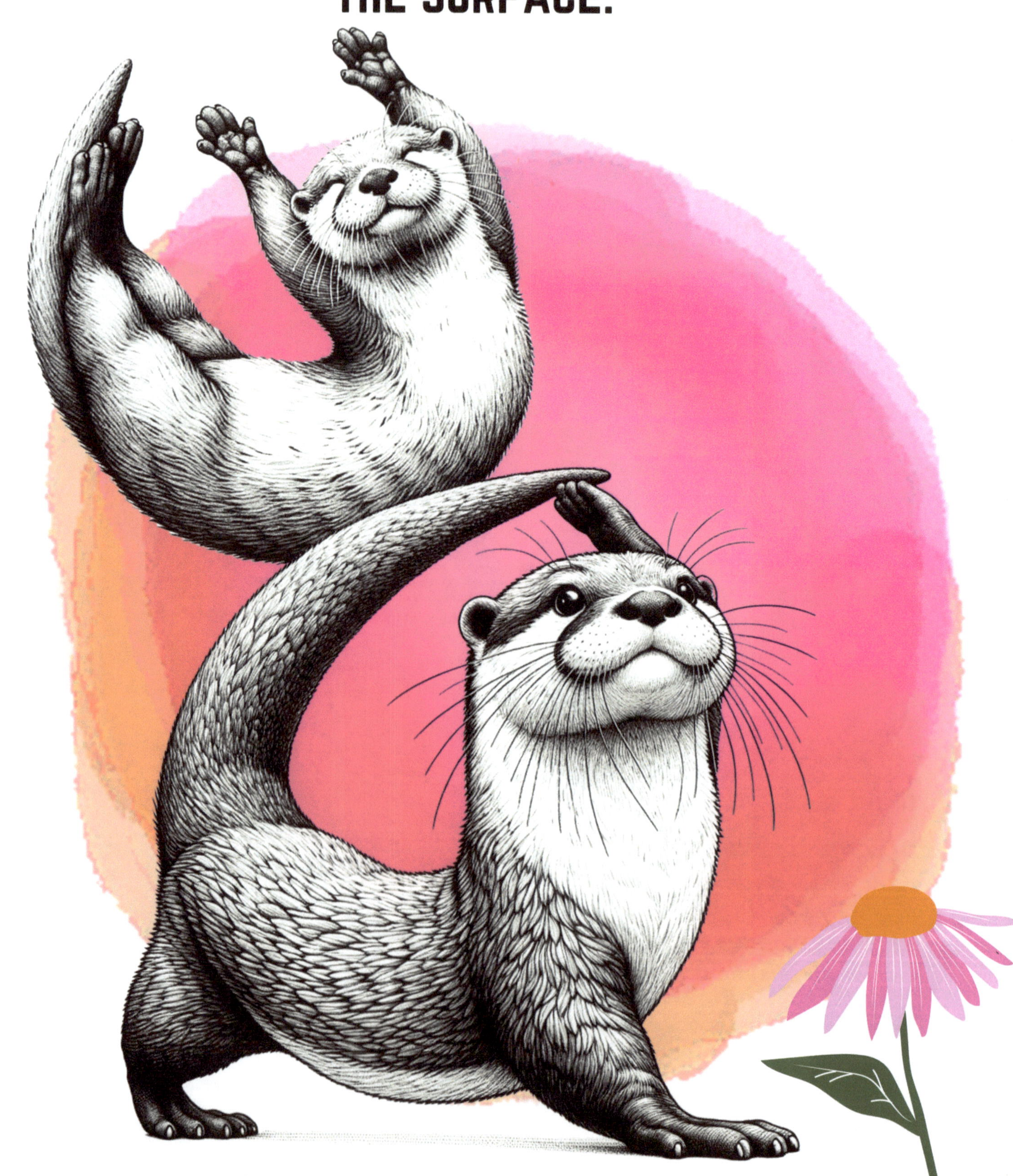

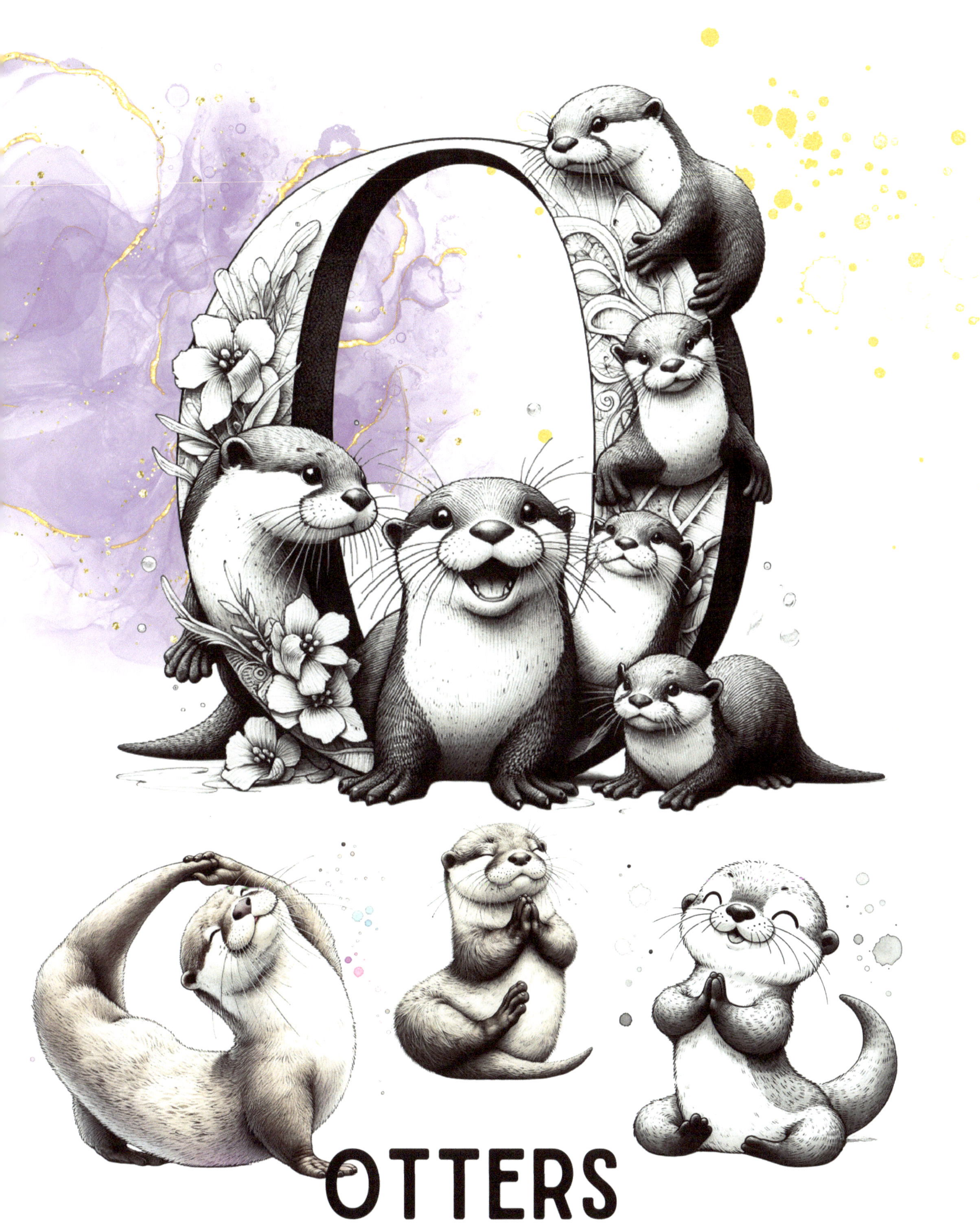

OTTERS

PORCUPINE MEANS "QUILL PIG". HOWEVER, THEY ARE NOT PIGS AT ALL. PORCUPINES ARE AMONG THE LARGEST RODENTS ON EARTH.

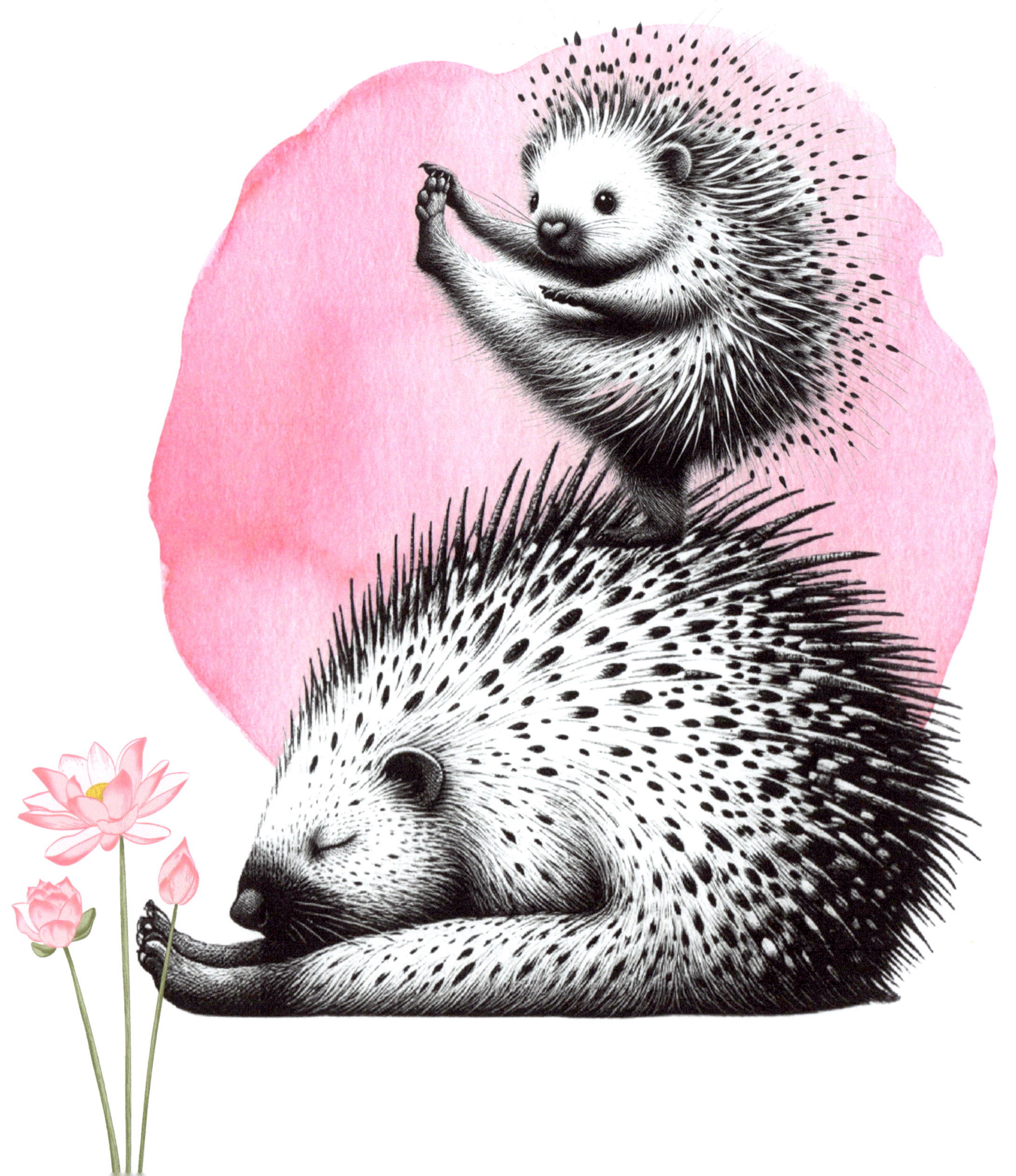

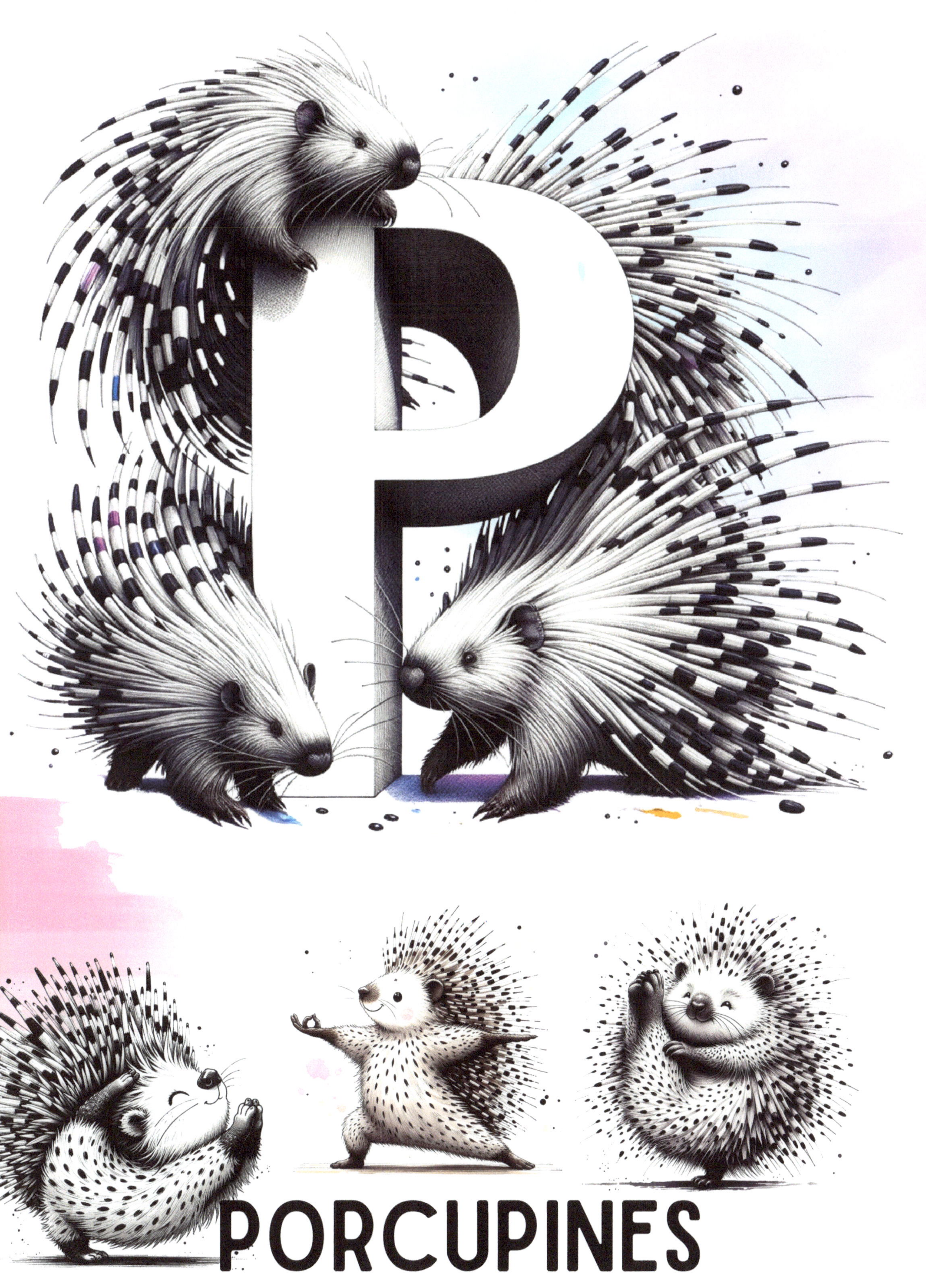

P
PORCUPINES

QUAILS ARE OFTEN VERY SHY BIRDS. IT IS MORE COMMON TO HEAR THEIR UNIQUE GRUNTING HUMMING SOUND THAN IT IS TO SEE THEM.

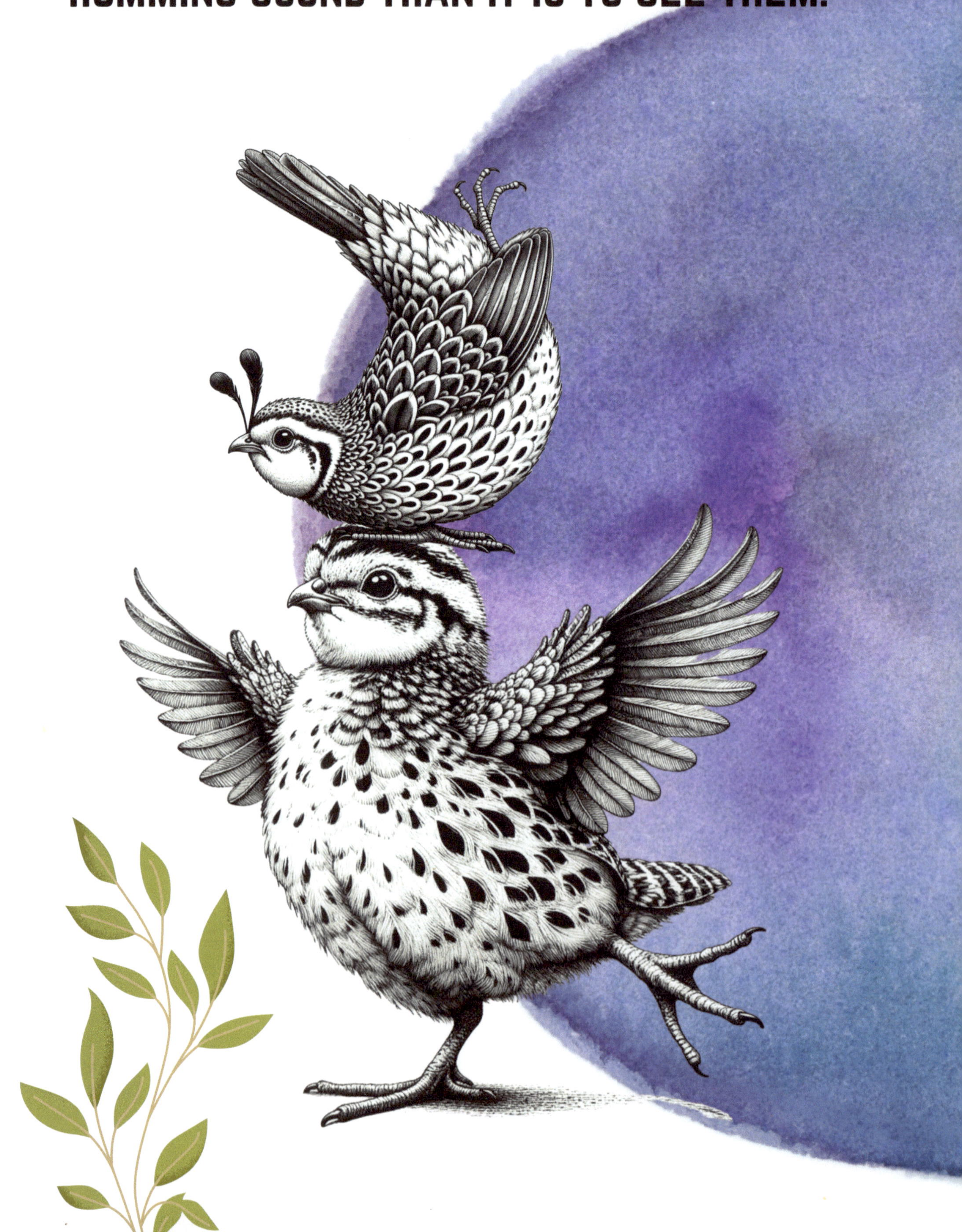

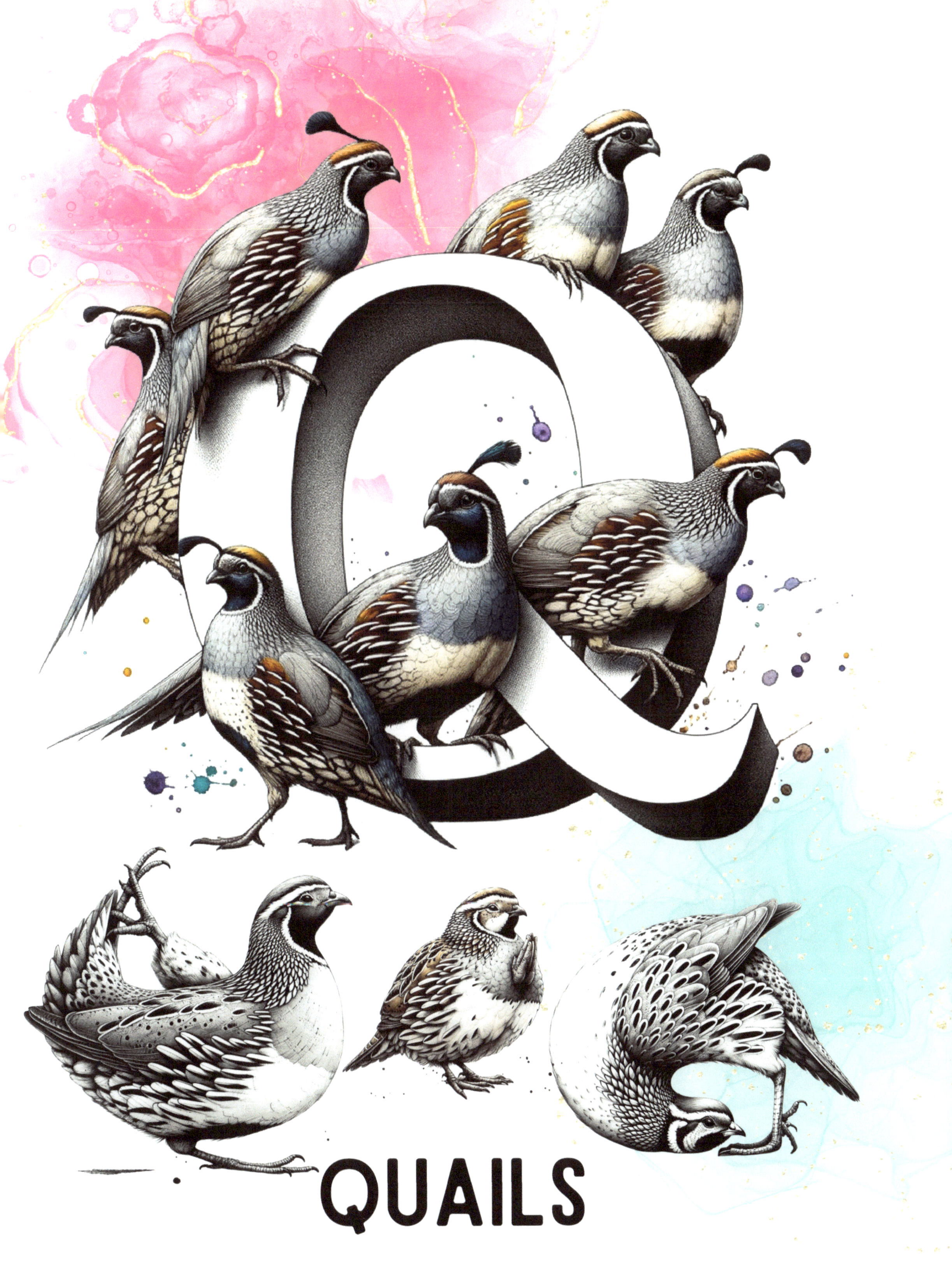

QUAILS

WE OFTEN THINK OF RATTLENSAKES AS BEING DANGEROUS PREDATORS. IN REALITY, THEY ARE ACTUALLY IN DANGER OF BECOMING PREY TO MANY ANIMALS INCLUDING EAGLES, OWLS, HAWKS, FOXES AND COYOTES.

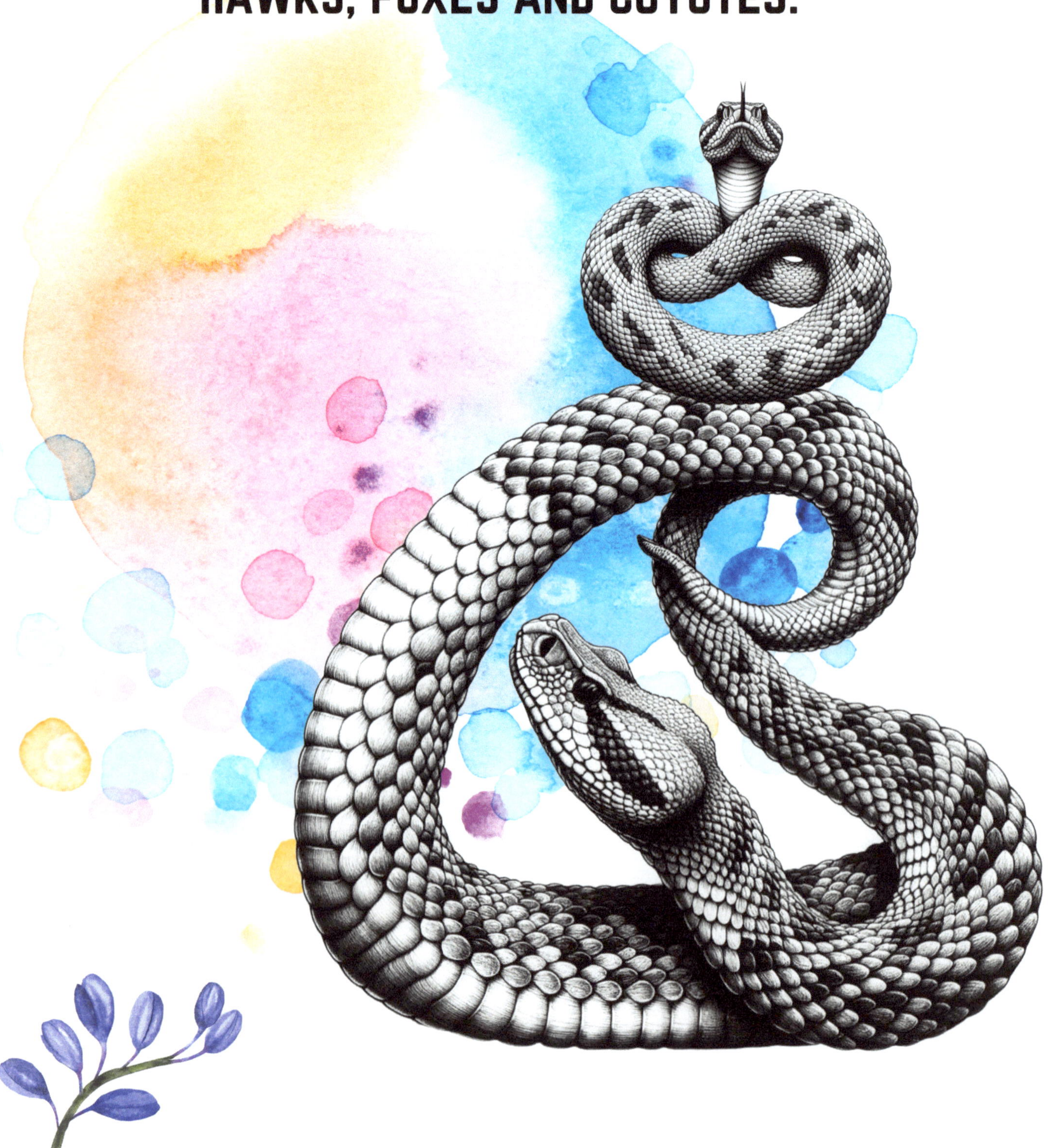

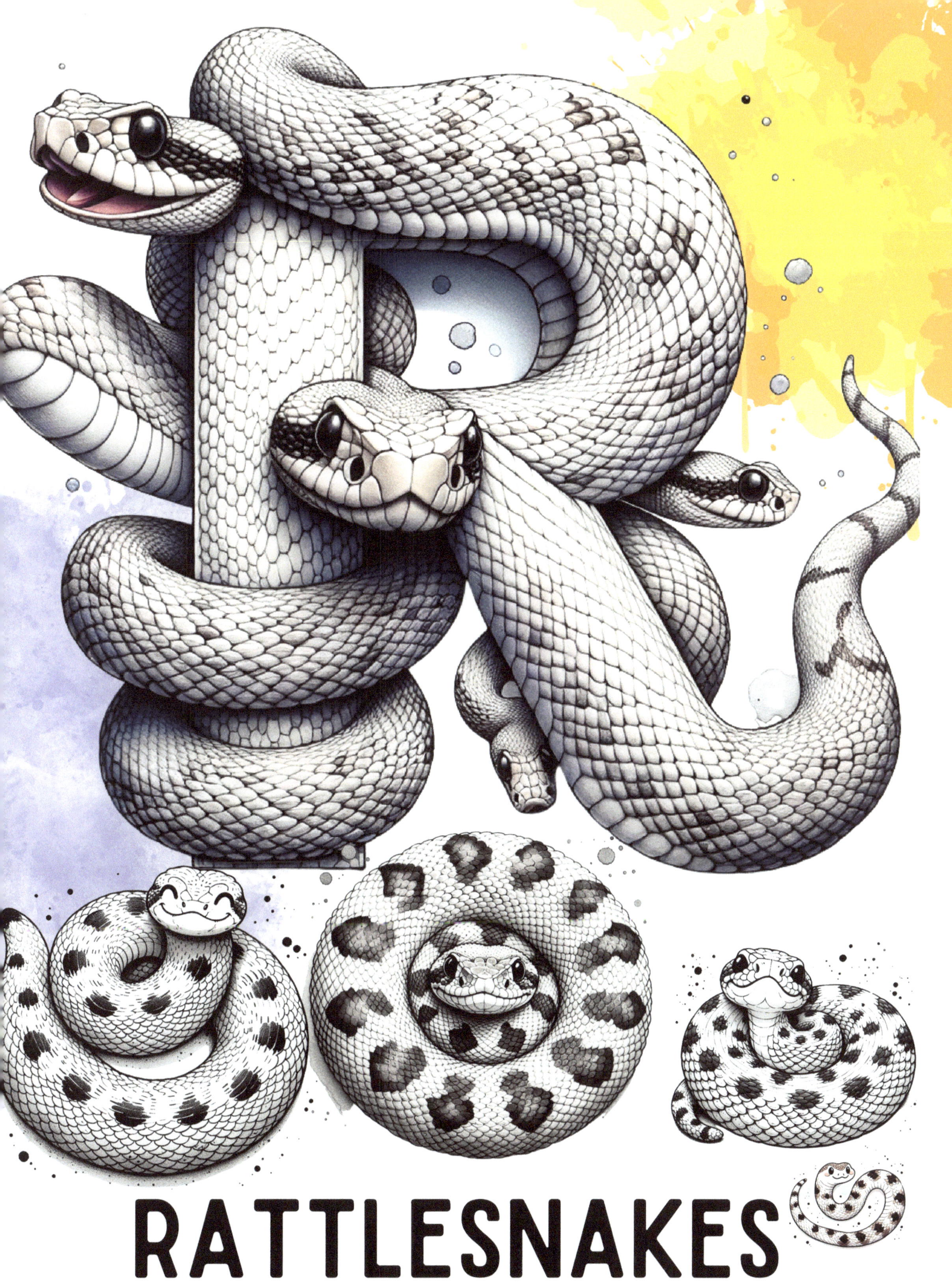

RATTLESNAKES

SEAHORSES DON'T LOOK LIKE TYPICAL FISH, BUT THEY ARE ACTUALLY CLASSIFIED AS FISH. THEY CAN EAT UP TO 3,000 TINY BRINE SHRIMP A DAY.

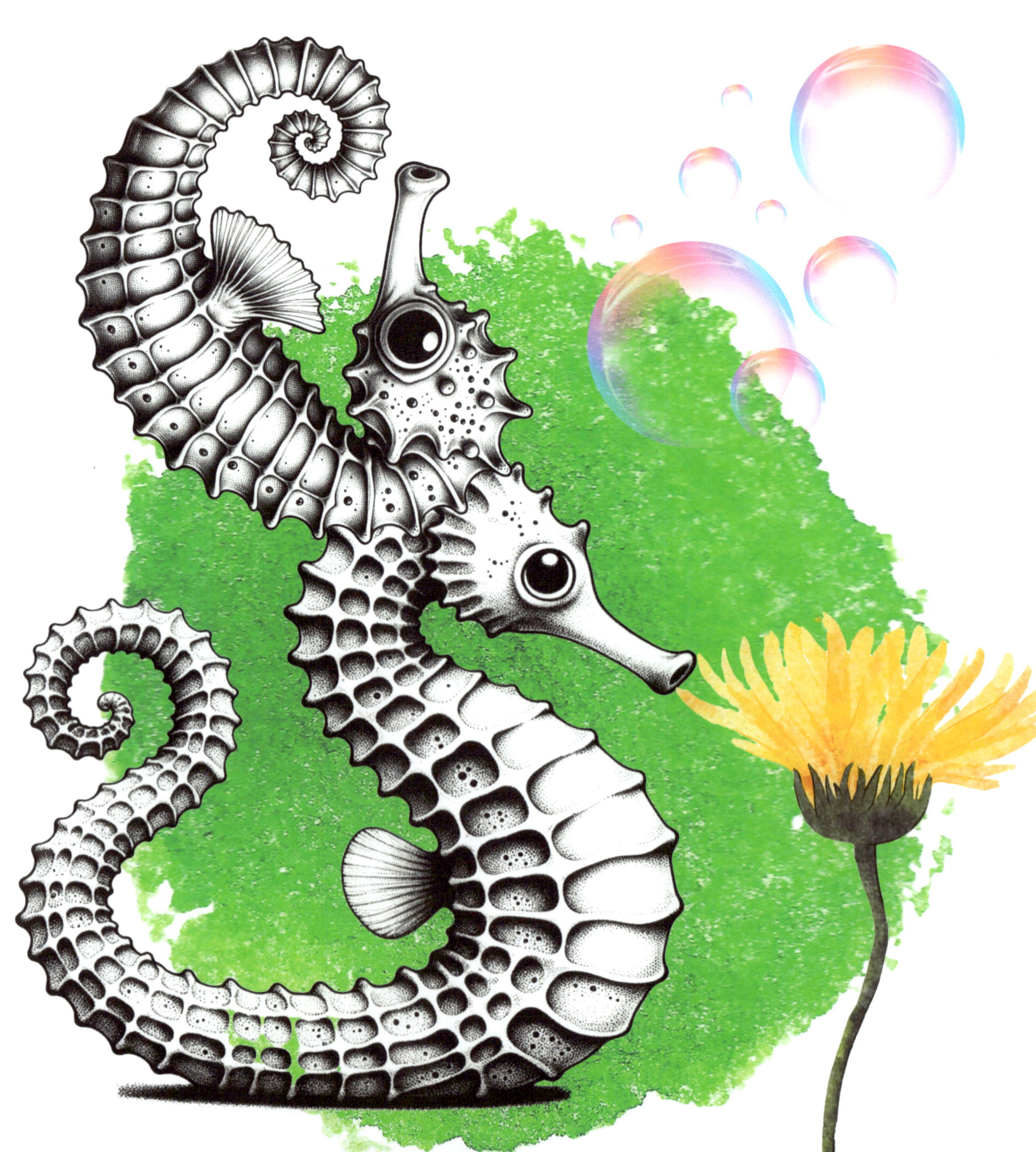

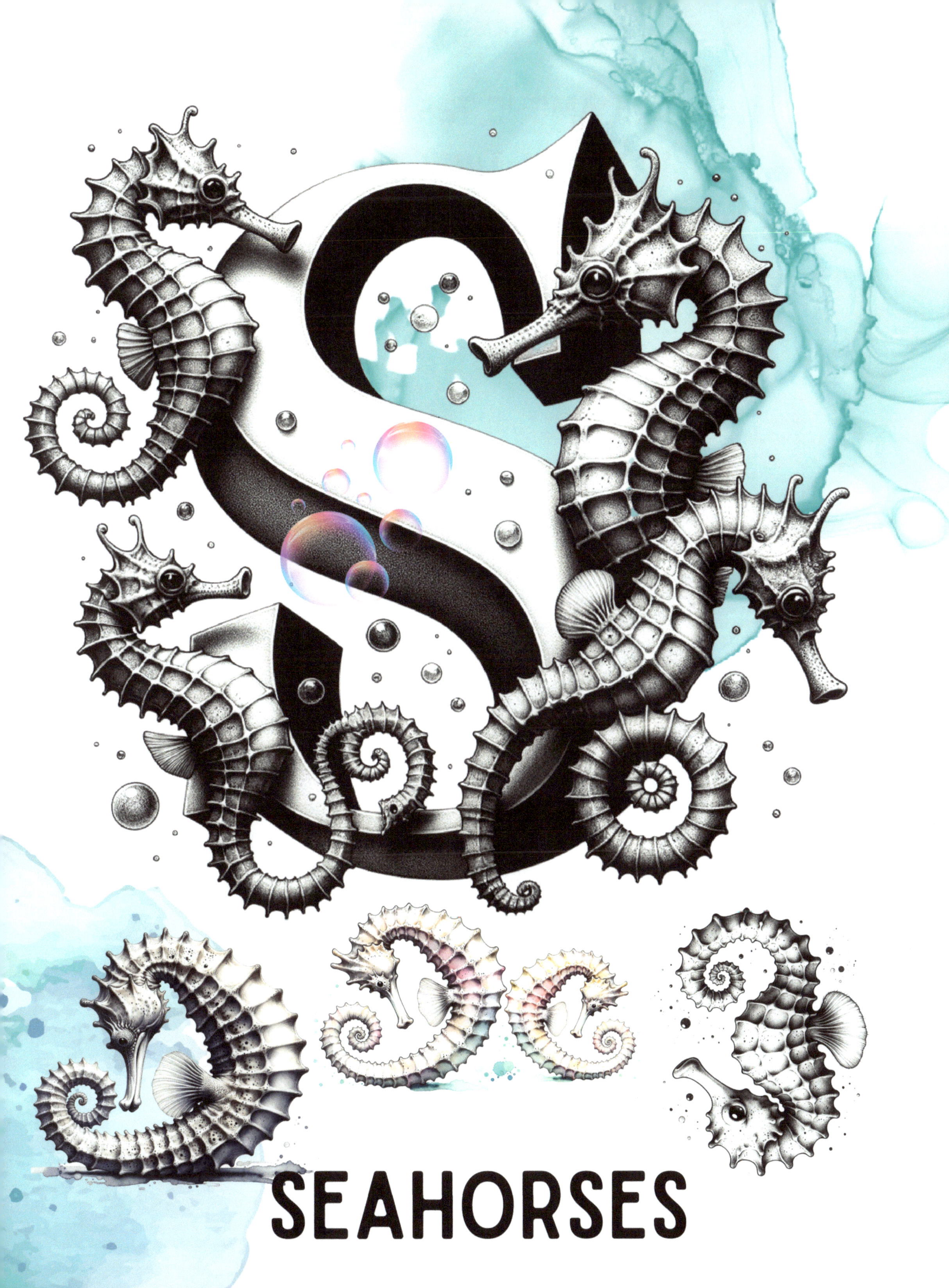

SEAHORSES

TURTLES ARE AMONG THE LONGEST-EXISTING ANIMALS ON EARTH. THEY HAVE BEEN AROUND SINCE THE DAYS OF DINOSAURS. SOME TYPES OF TURTLES CAN LIVE OVER 100 YEARS.

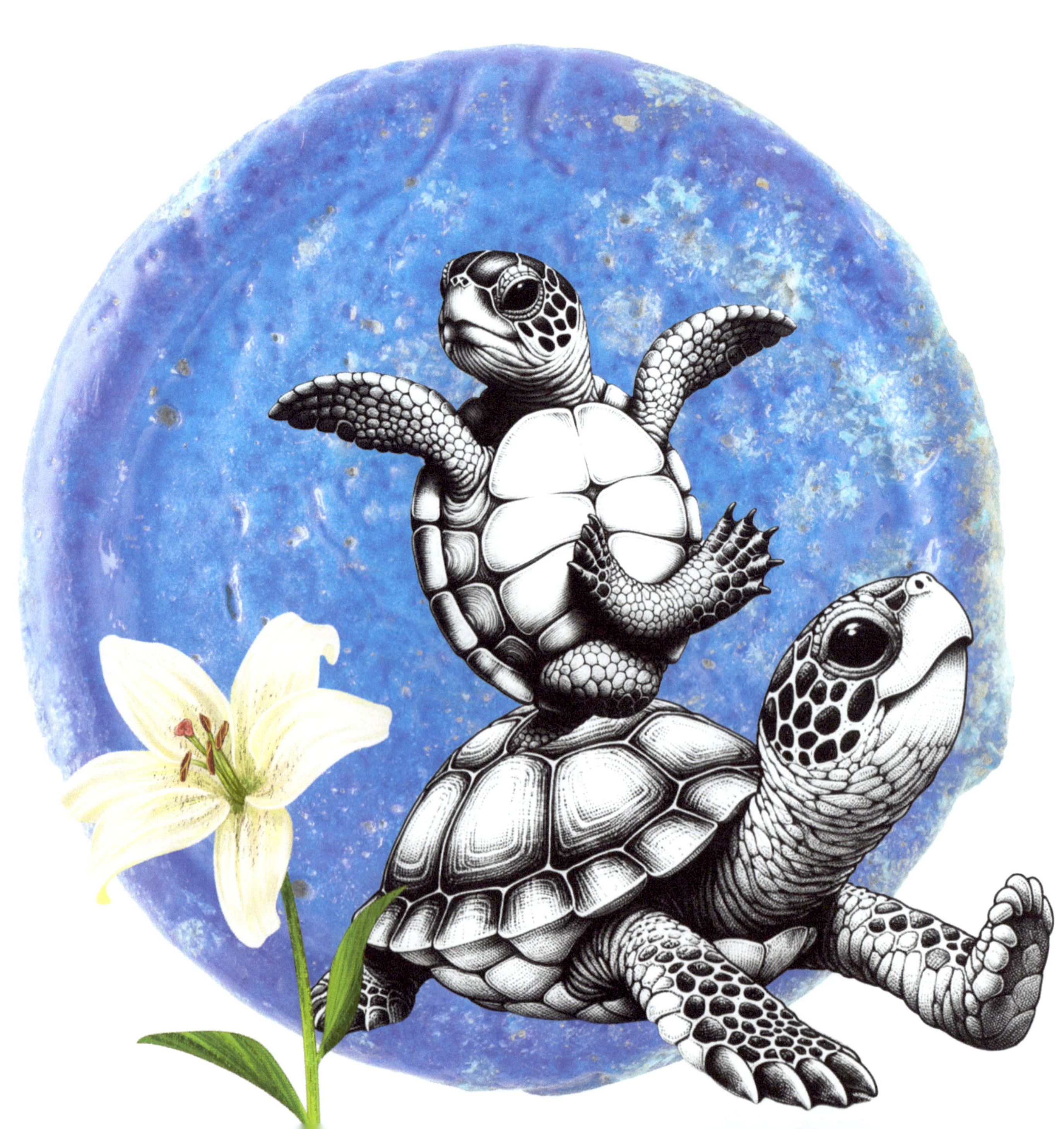

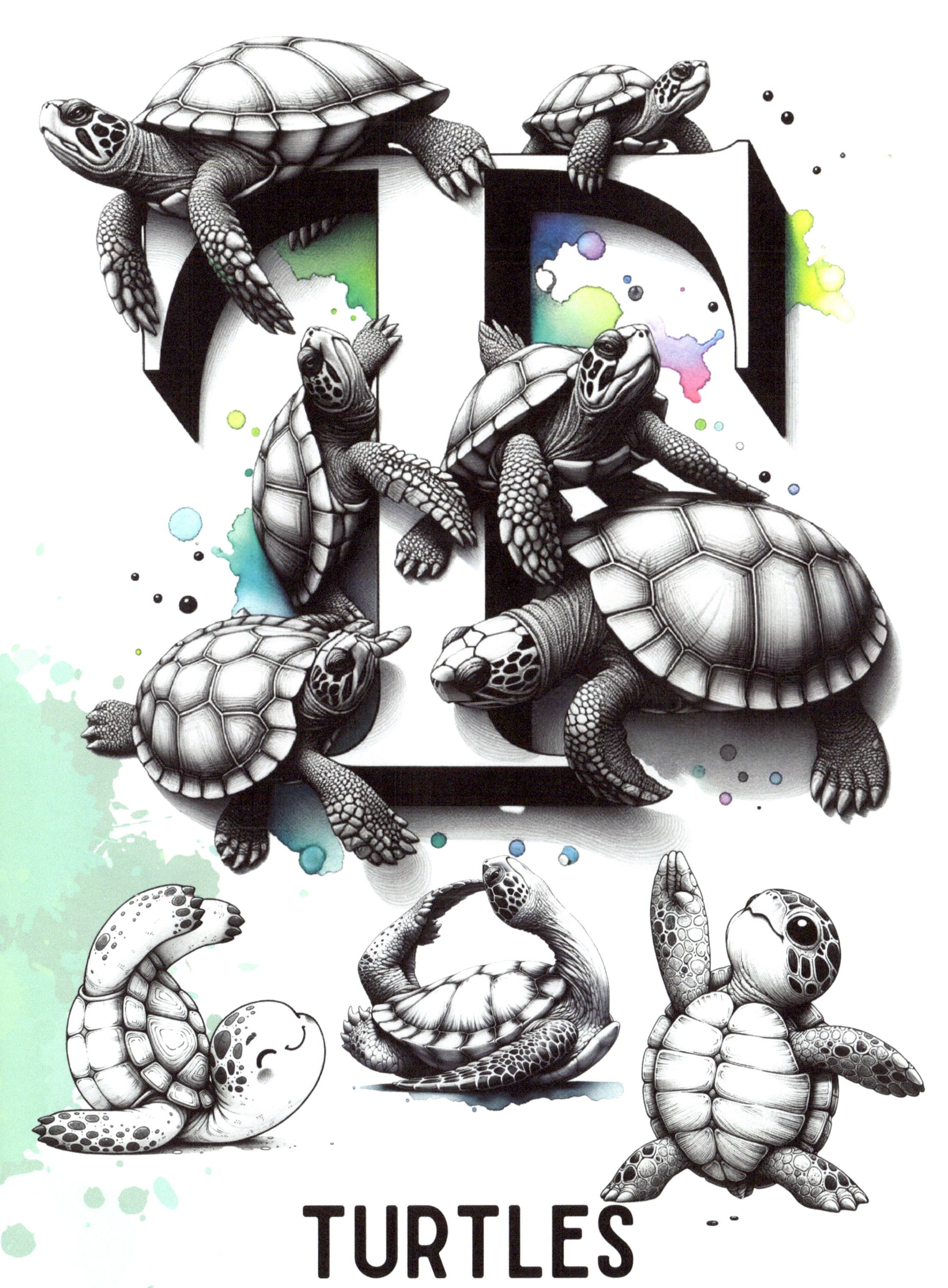

TURTLES

URCHINS HAVE HUNDREDS OF TINY FEET TO HELP THEM MOVE SLOWLY ALONG ROCKS UNDERWATER. URCHINS HAVE NO BONES. INSTEAD, THEY HAVE A HARD SHELL.

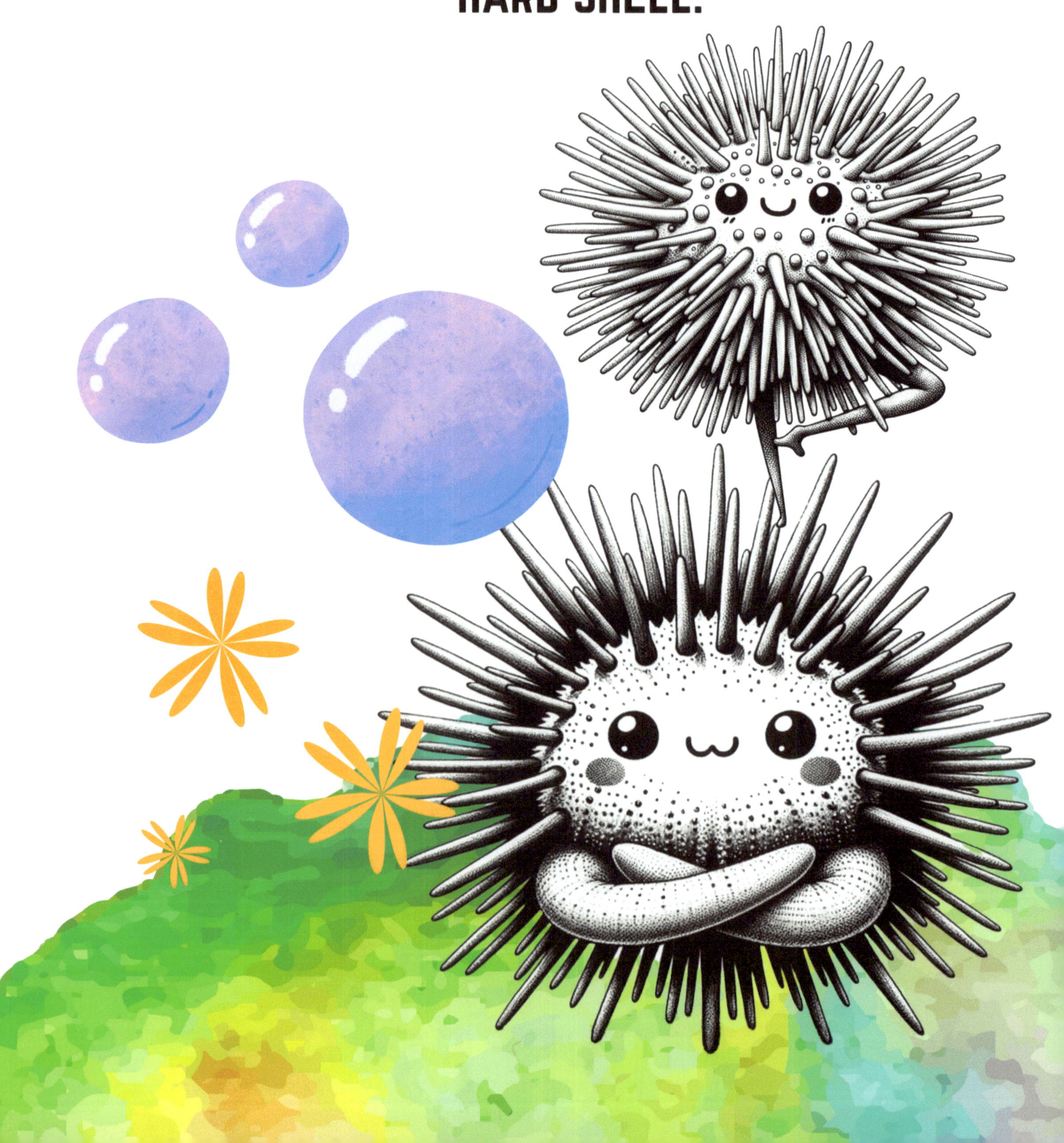

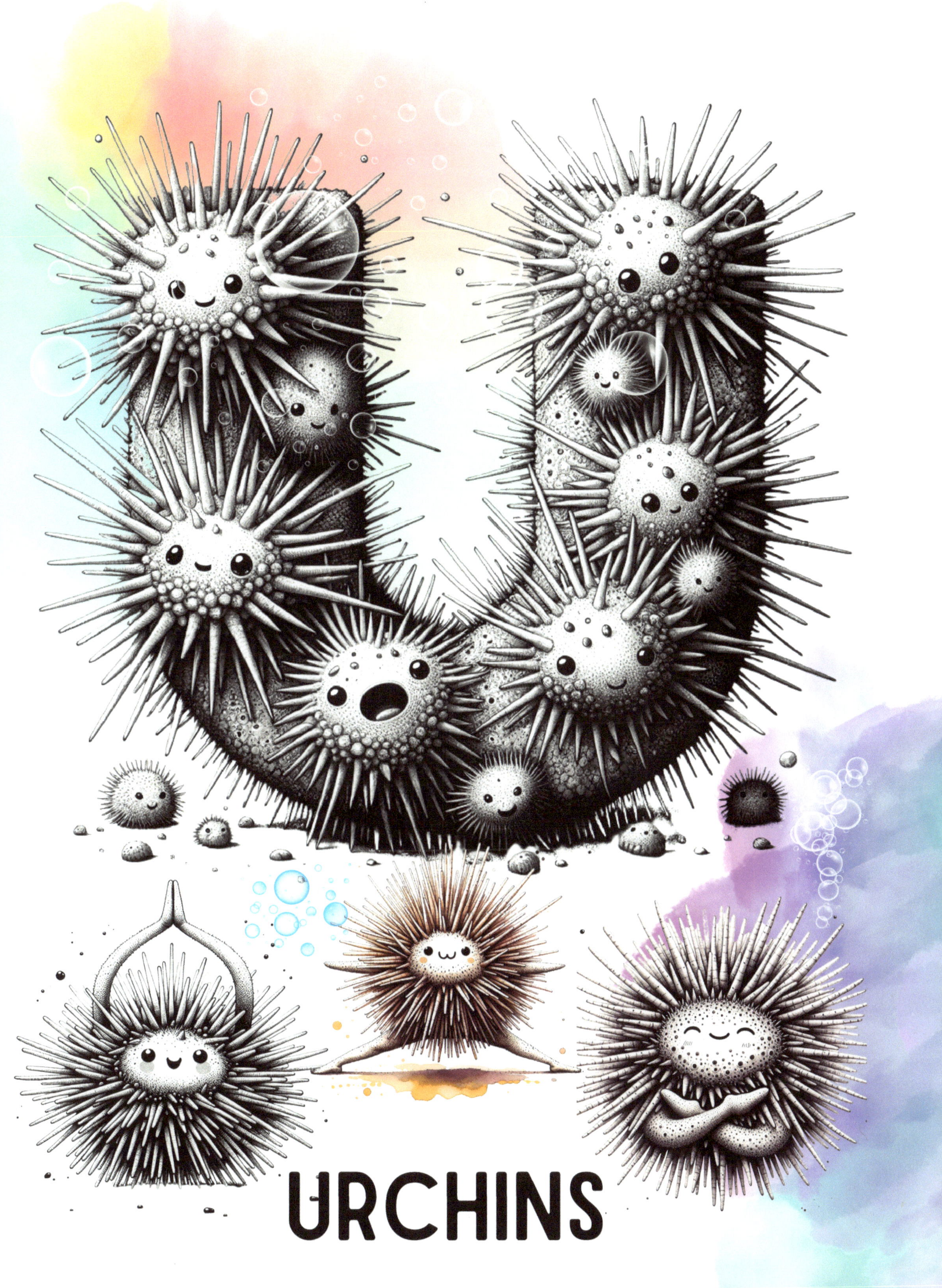

URCHINS

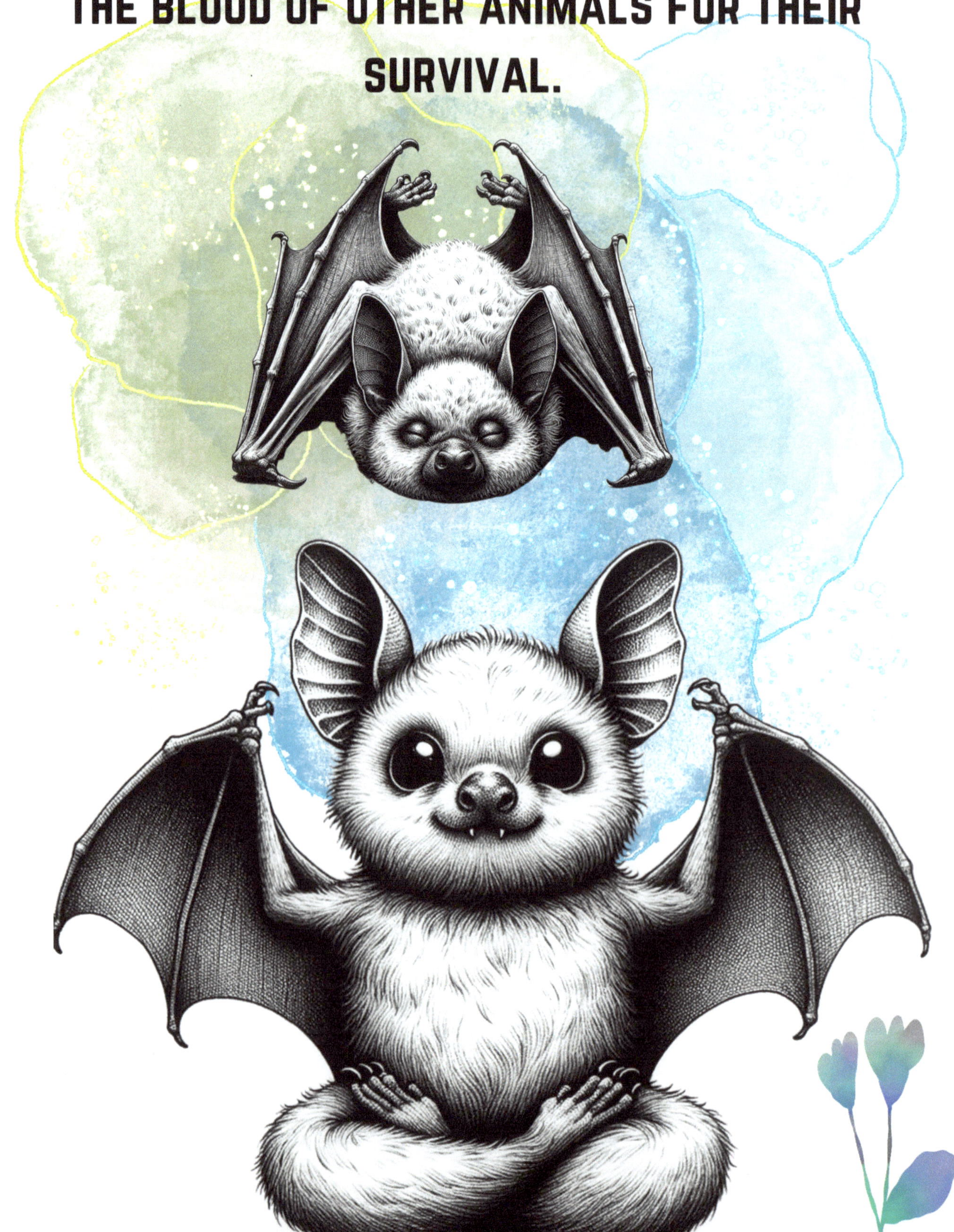
Out of 1,400 species of bats on Earth, only three species are considered "Vampire bats". This means they rely on consuming the blood of other animals for their survival.

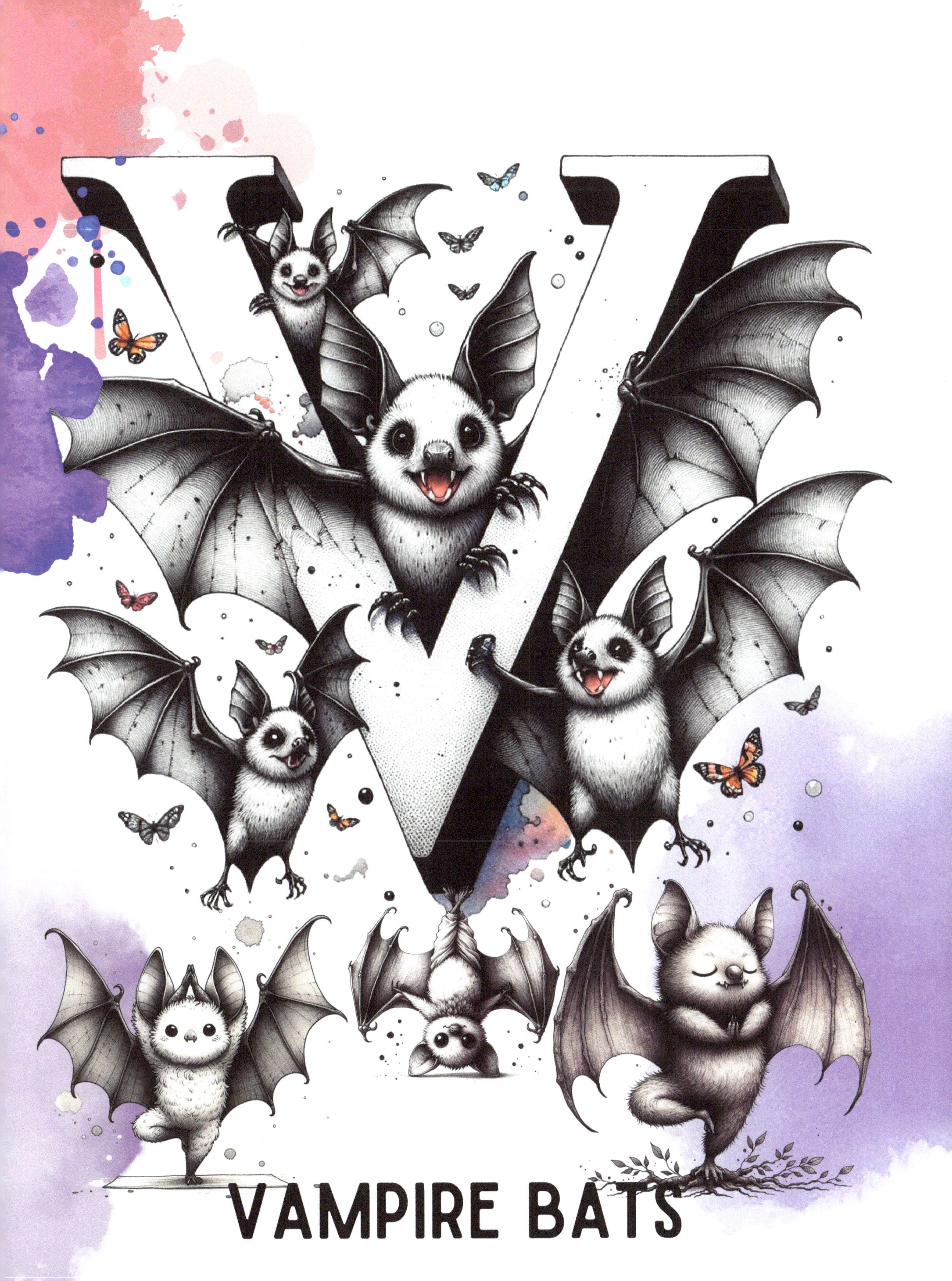

VAMPIRE BATS

WALRUS TUSKS CAN BE UP TO 3 FEET LONG. THEY USE THE TUSKS TO PULL THEMSELVES OUT OF THE WATER, TO CUT THROUGH ICE AND TO DEFEND THEMSELVES.

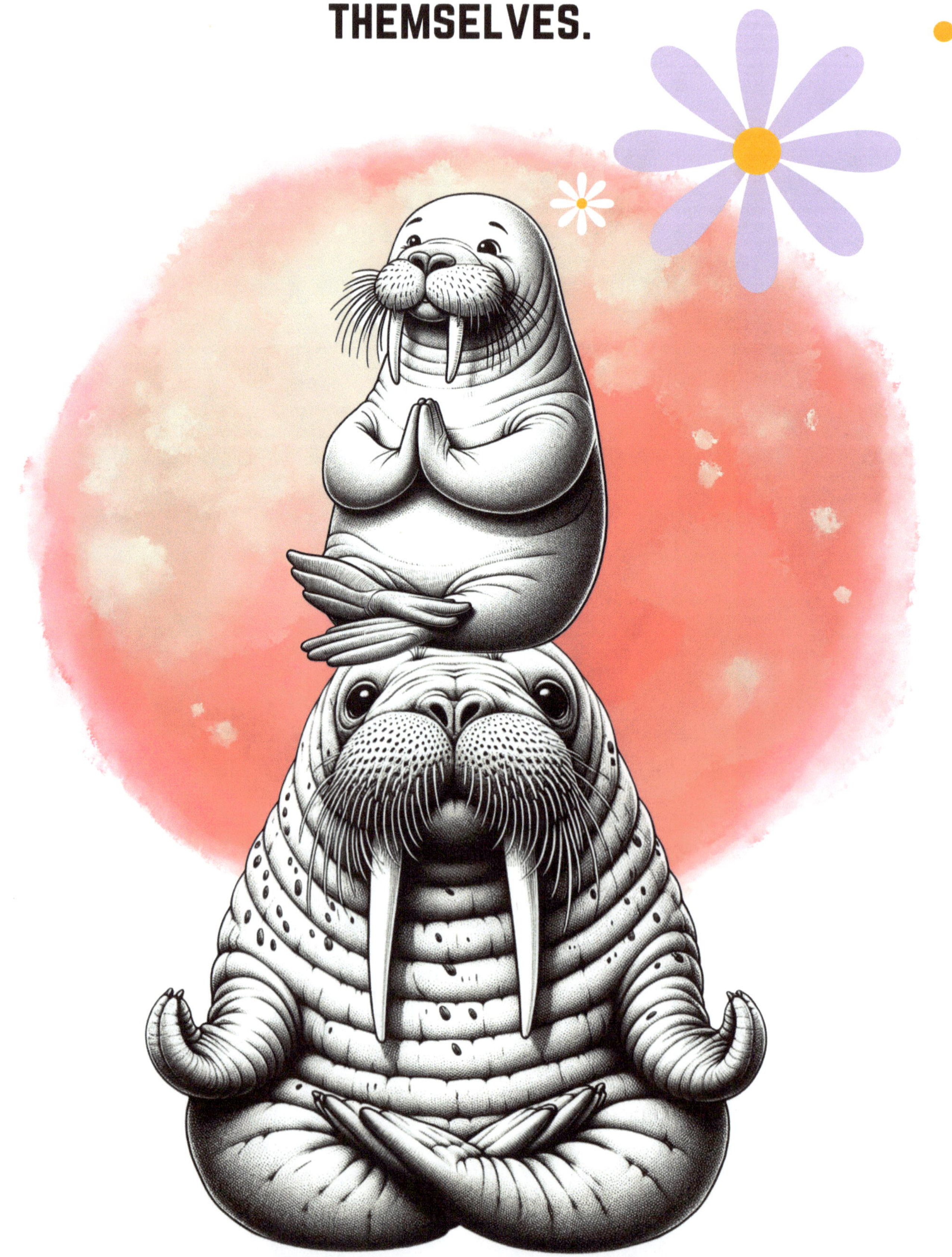

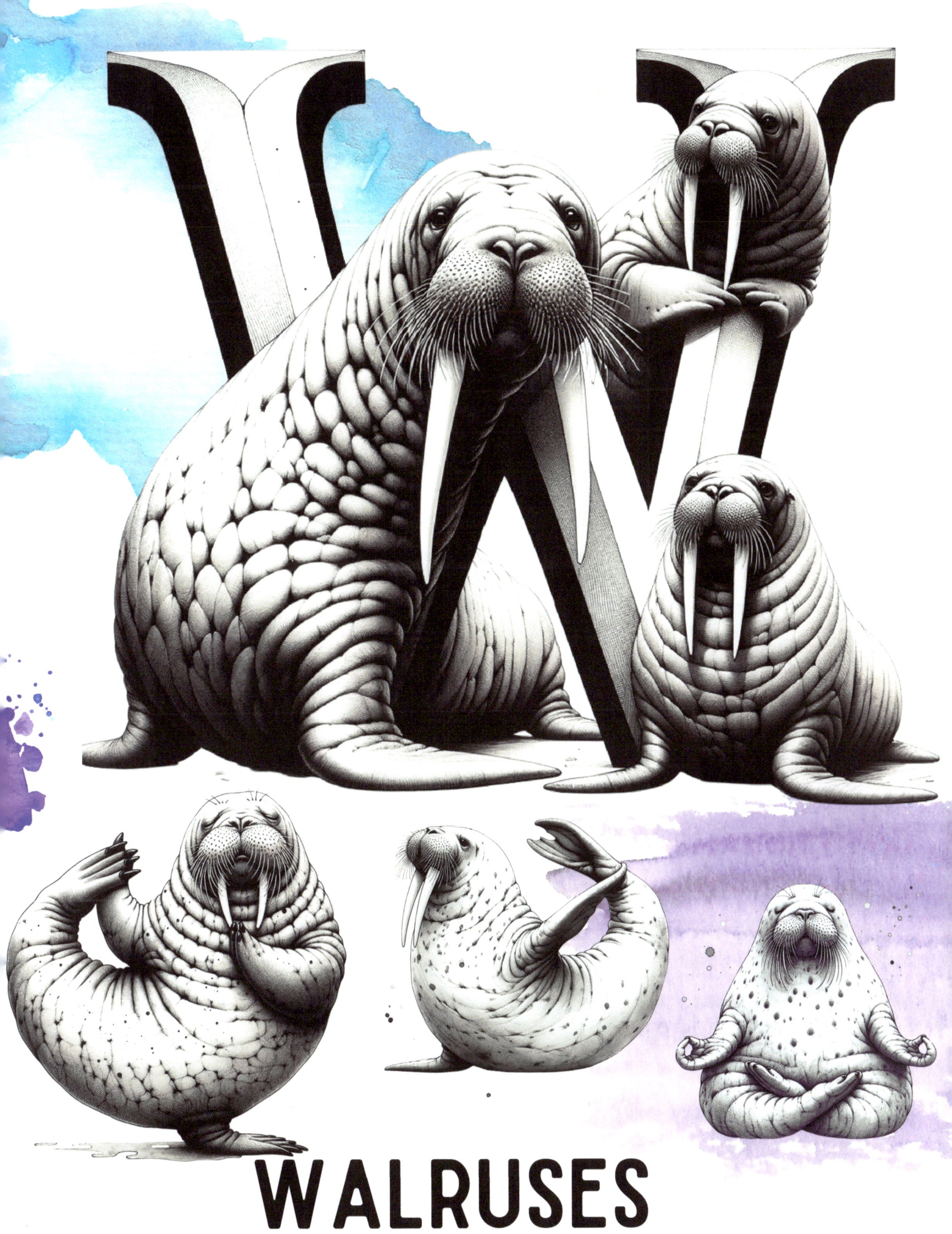

WALRUSES

Sadly, the Xerces Blue butterfly is extinct. The last one was seen in 1943, on the California Coast near San Francisco. They are only in this book because there aren't many animals whose names start with the letter X!

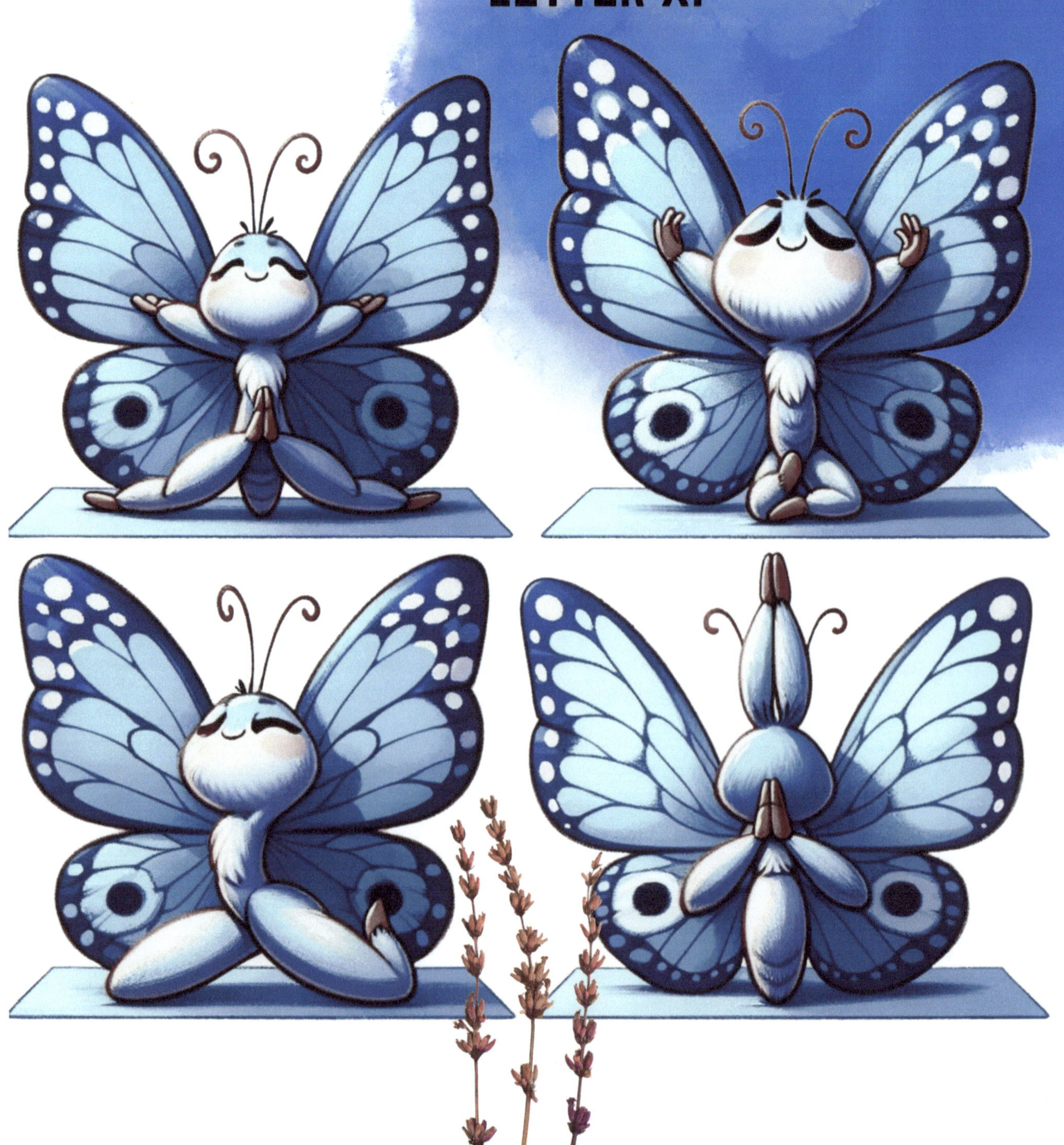

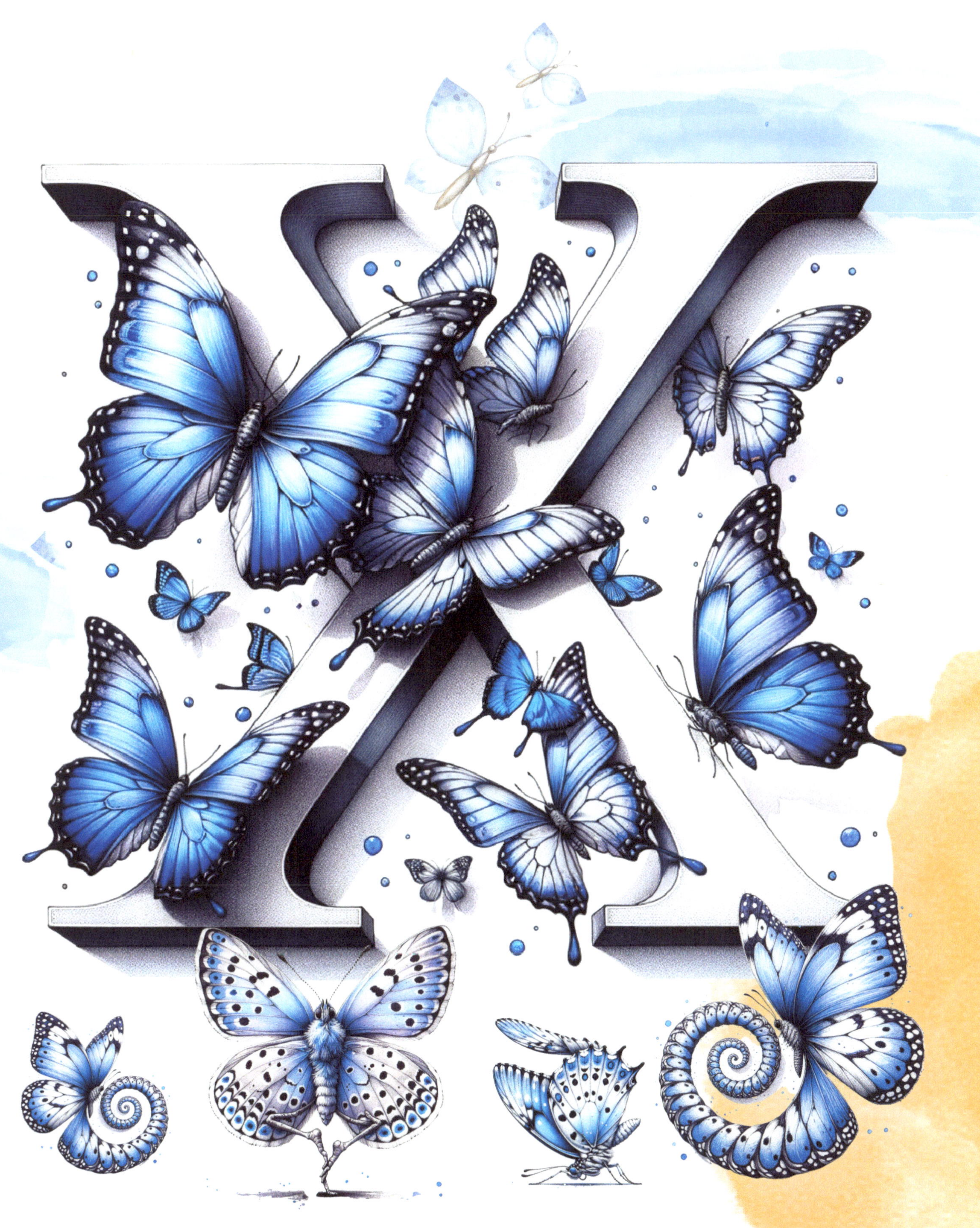

XERCES BLUE BUTTERFLIES

Yaks can live at very high altitudes and are often used as sources of milk in the mountainous regions of Asia.

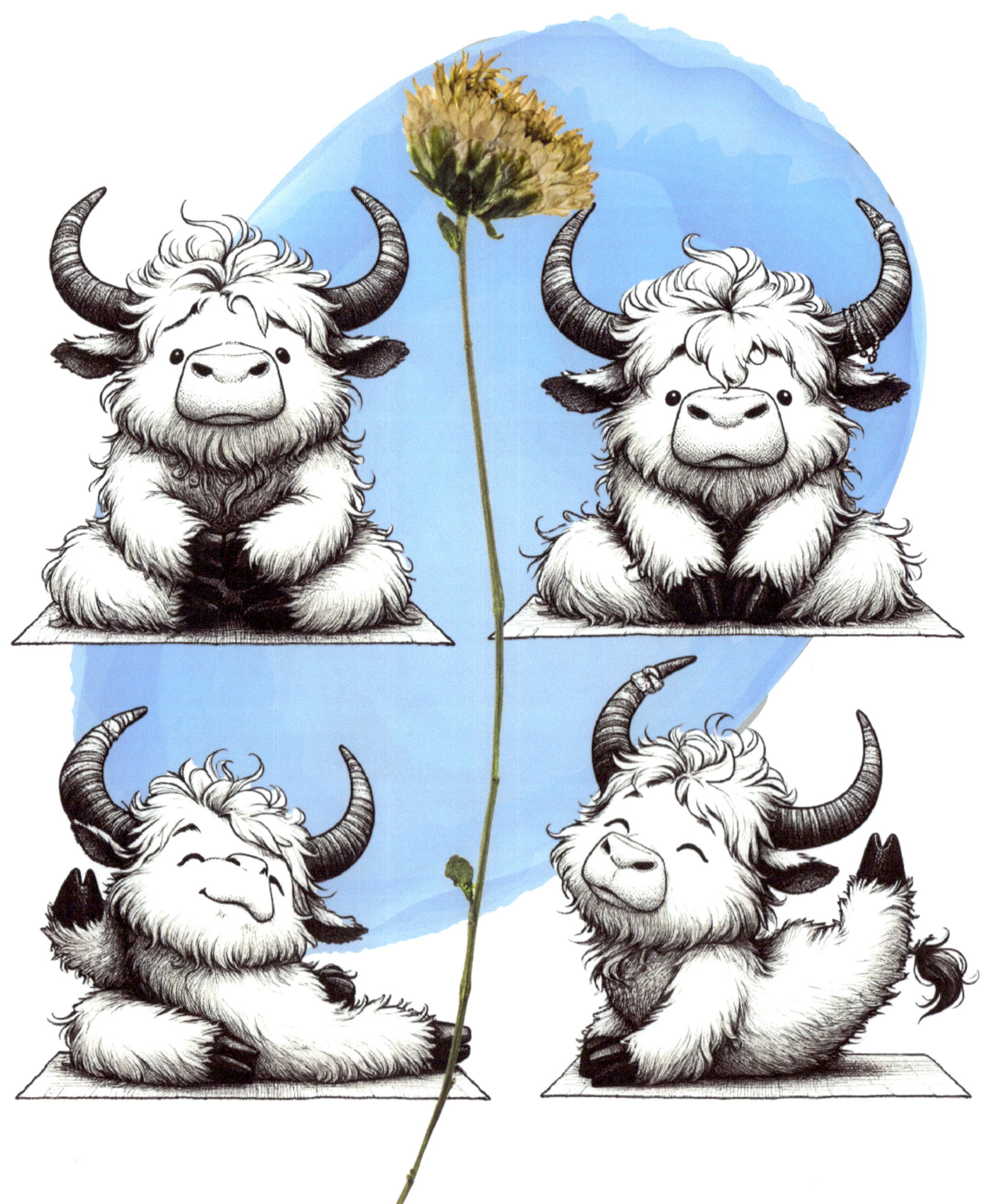

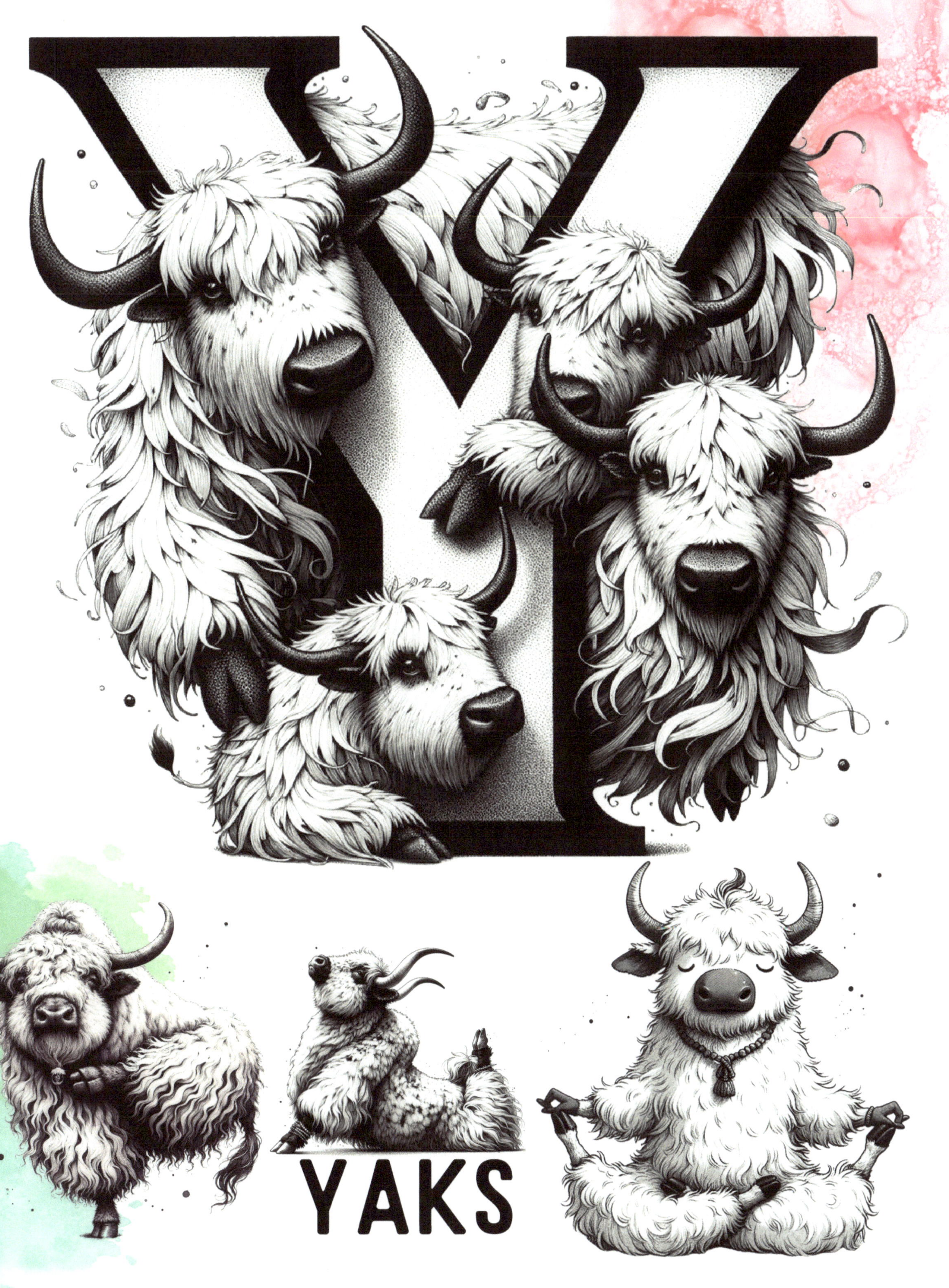

YAKS

ZigZag Salamanders are quite small, usually only about 3 inches long. They are capable of living for over ten years in captivity (when kept as pets)!

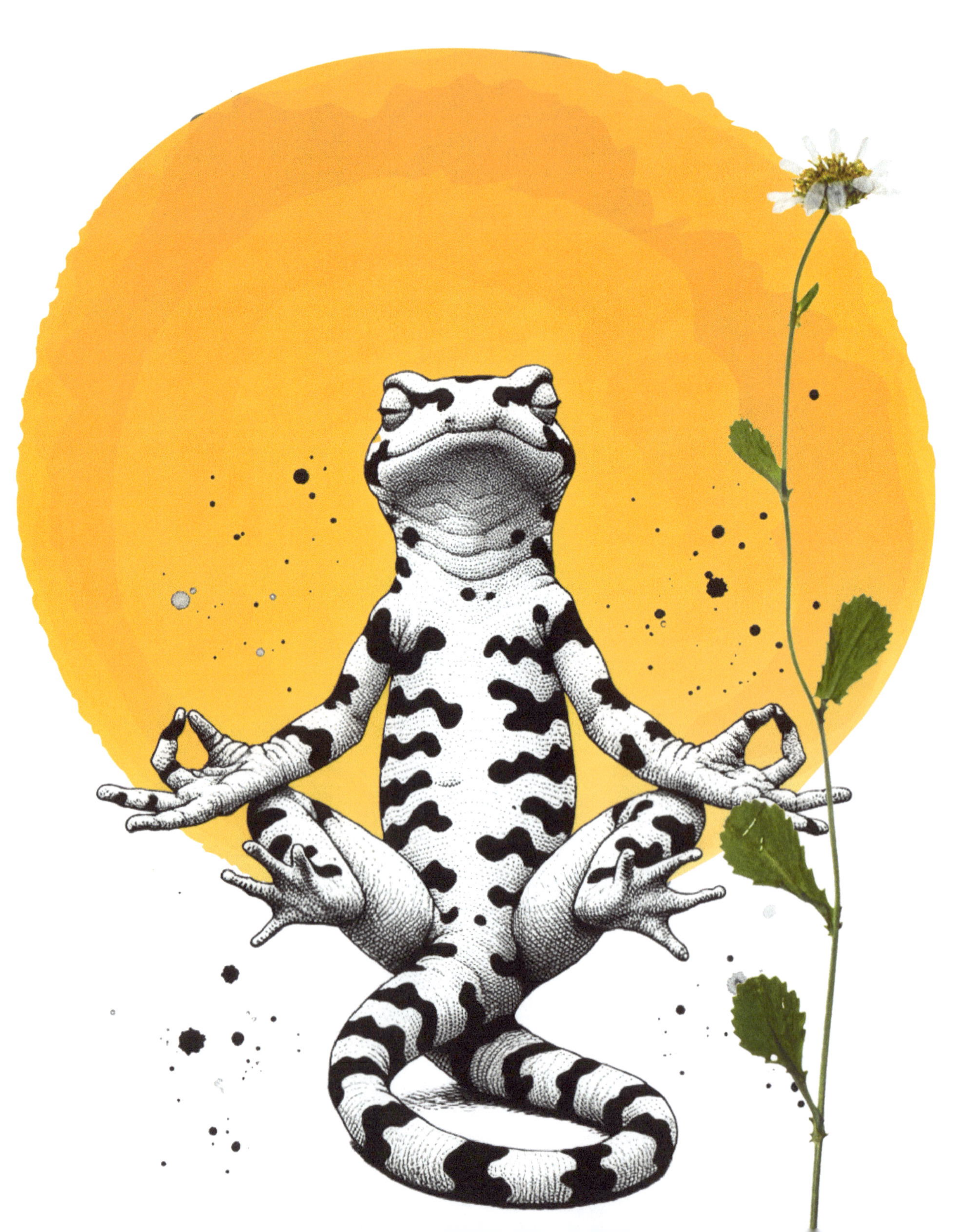

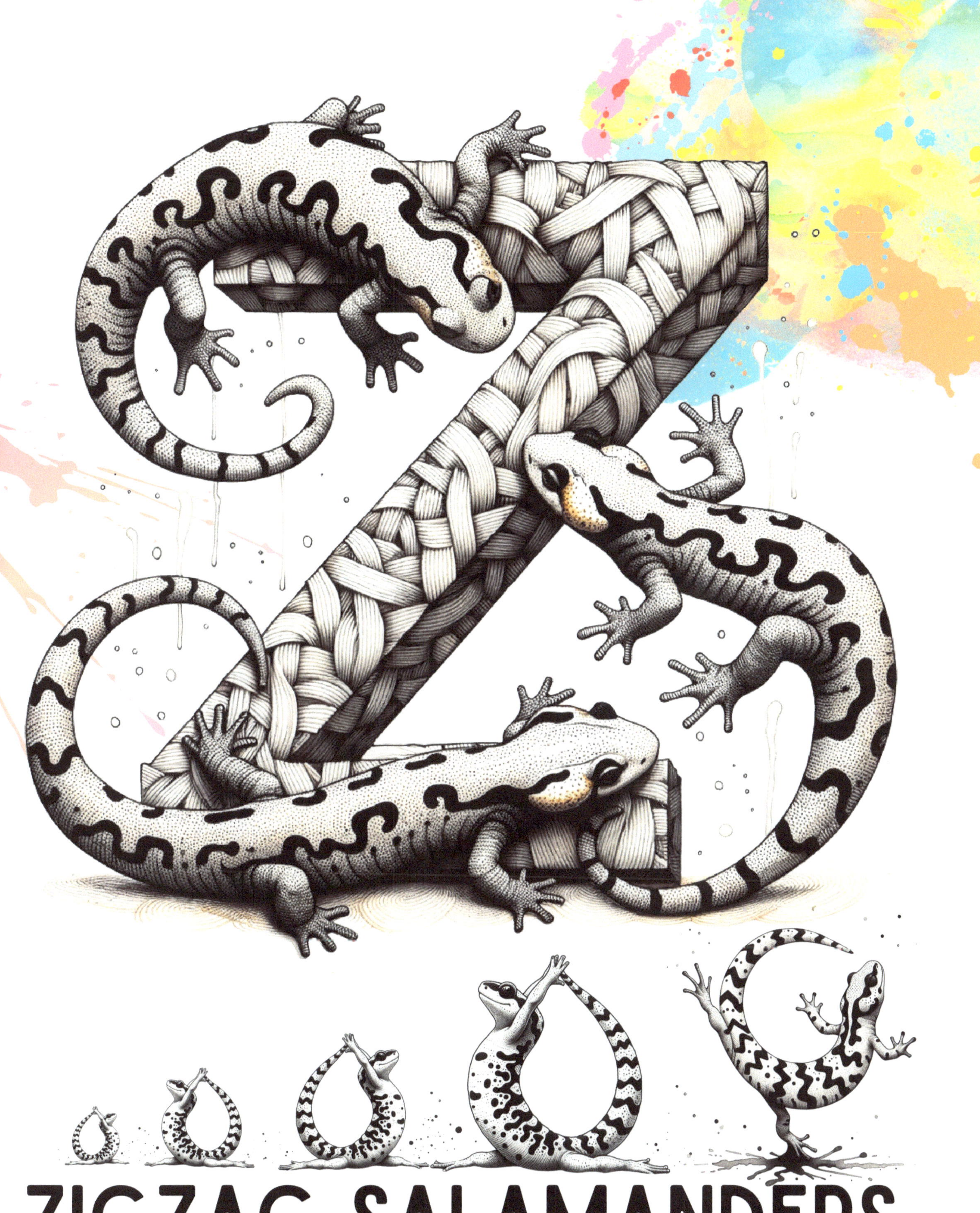

ZIGZAG SALAMANDERS

We hope you have enjoyed this book
And all the creatures, A to Z -
We only wish there were more letters
To bring delight to thee!

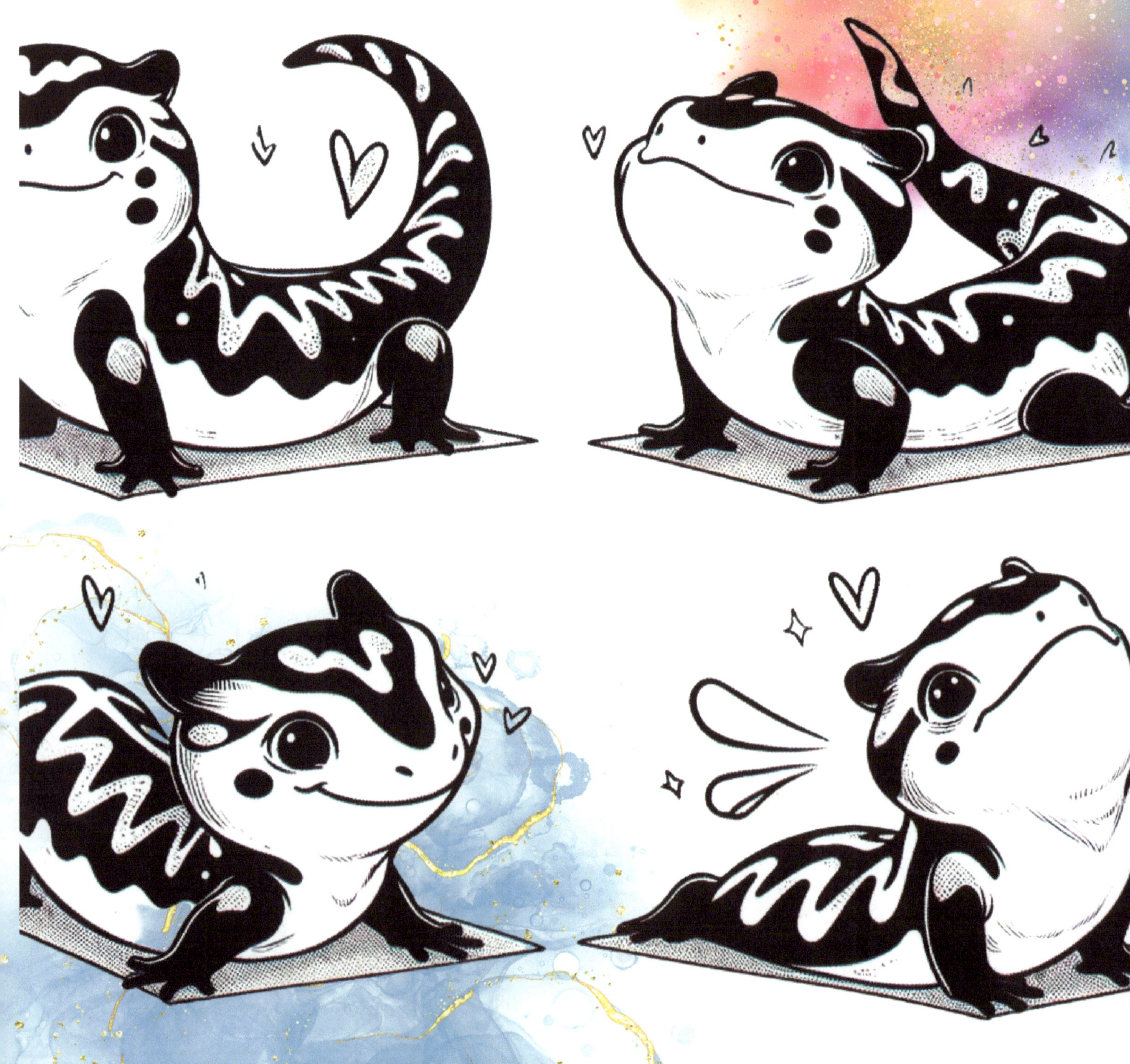

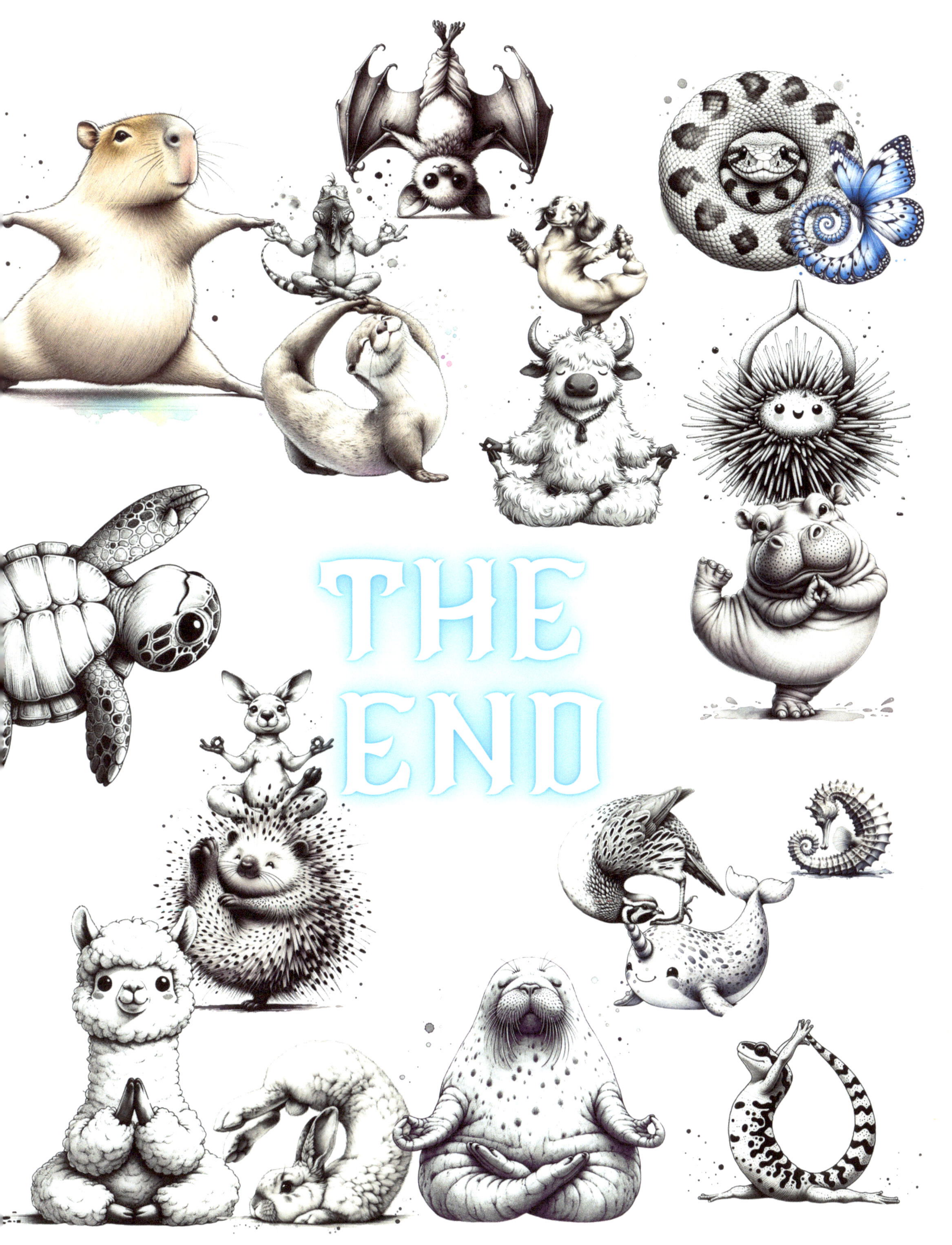
THE
END

www.ingramcontent.com/pod-product-compliance
Lightning Source LLC
Chambersburg PA
CBHW040137240726
48664CB00002B/520